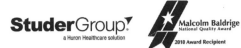

Healing Physician Burnout

Diagnosing, Preventing, and Treating

Quint Studer
in collaboration with
George Ford, MD

Published by:
Fire Starter Publishing
350 W. Cedar Street
Pensacola, FL 32502
Phone: 866-354-3473
Fax: 850-332-5117
www.firestarterpublishing.com

ISBN: 978-1-622-18020-2

Library of Congress Control Number: 2015945172

Printed in the United States of America

This book is dedicated to all the physicians past, present, and future who have been, and continue to be, the lifeblood of healthcare.

TABLE OF CONTENTS

Preface:

Now Is the Time

This is a book about burnout, but it's also a book about physician engagement and alignment. I find that burnout and engagement are opposite ends of the same spectrum. When physicians are engaged, they won't burn out, and when they do burnout, they're not engaged. And that's why this book is filled with tactics that health system leaders can use to proactively engage physicians to avoid burnout—as well as to ensure that everyone is working toward the same goals. Physicians deserve a positive work environment. This book is about helping to make that happen while shining a bright light on the burnout causes.

Many of the tactics in this book have been around for a while. And yet, despite sincere efforts, many physicians still are frustrated in their work. One might wonder why that is. Why, if those tactics are good and have been around for some time, aren't they being practiced more consistently? My theory is that previously the time wasn't right for making physician engagement and alignment work. Now, the time *is* right.

I bring this up early on because I don't want anyone to read this book and think healthcare system leaders have not thought about physician engagement and alignment, or that it has not been a priority. It has been. In fact, in the late 1980s or perhaps it was the early 1990s, I remember reading a book on the need to create fully vertically integrated healthcare systems. However, the payment system in many ways just did not support hospital and physician alignment.

At What's Right in Healthcare®, Studer Group's annual conference, every year a few healthcare system leaders present on physician engagement and share their physician satisfaction survey results and steps they've taken to improve results. However, obviously, the tactics these leaders describe have not been implemented as well as everyone would like. Why? In the simplest terms, it's because the healthcare payment system had always been set up to make physician and health system alignment very difficult.

So what has changed? For one thing, value-based purchasing has become a reality. For another, there are many, many more physicians employed by healthcare systems than there used to be. Now these physicians are part of the system in a way that they weren't before. Even the ones who are not employed by a healthcare system will be connected to the healthcare system through an accountable care organization, or managed care contracting, or population health management, or medical homes. All of a sudden, we all have skin in the game.

In the past, that wasn't true. One might read a physician satisfaction survey, and, of course, *want* to get everybody engaged, but the payment system would sometimes create conflicting goals. So we had that very difficult situation where we had to decide: What do we collaborate in and what do we compete with? (The truth is you can run a good healthcare system and still have collaboration and competition in the group. However, it is very difficult and time consuming.) We even had situations where it was counter-productive to work together. As reimbursement was reduced, trying to figure out who does what (procedures, surgery, tests) and where they do it became a jousting match.

So what we found in the past was that even though the health systems had access to tools and tactics that could reduce physician burnout—and although all truly wanted to be successful—creating the consistency needed to optimize the tactics was not easy. Now with many organizations being more fully integrated, with increased employment of physicians, with accountable care organizations, with population health, with shared risk formulas, suddenly everybody is on the same page, or soon will be.

Physicians are highly intelligent. It doesn't take them long to figure out "Now that I'm working on the same team, I'm now locked into the success of the healthcare system. If the healthcare system is struggling financially and operationally, that will impact my potential and my compensation. And my own performance will impact the health of the organization." In other words, the physician's future and the healthcare system's future are one and the same.

We've always said that physicians need a strong healthcare system, but now we mean it in a deeper way. Physicians need a strong healthcare system psychologically because they want their patients to have good care. But now they also need it to be successful because of their own job security. Their ability to provide good care to patients will rest on the health of the healthcare organization. They need equipment; they need supplies; they may need an upgraded facility and new patient access points. All of that depends on the healthcare system being a very strong one and everyone—physicians, leaders, and staff—working together to make it strong.

As value-based purchasing is phased in and as physician productivity relative value units (RVUs) become less of a major element in the evaluation tool or compensation formula, the greater good starts winning. And as the greater good is captured, everyone benefits.

In the past, the external environment made it more difficult to get physicians aligned and engaged. Today, the external environment has actually created conditions in which the healthcare system, the physicians, and other providers are closer to being on the same page than ever before. This makes the ability to implement these tools and tactics not only a bit easier, but absolutely necessary and desired by not only the healthcare system, but also the physicians.

I want to make one other point as well: Right now there is a lot of conversation happening around physician leadership and performance improvement. There is so much great work being done in these areas. For example, the American Medical Association (AMA) is zeroing in on these issues with its STEPS Forward™ series of educational modules for physicians. I applaud this effort and the efforts of other organizations doing similar work—however, that is not the focus of this book.

The focus of *Healing Physician Burnout* is on creating better work environments for physicians. For physicians to grow as leaders and learn vital new skills, they first have to be fully engaged and aligned. When health system leaders master the tactics in this book, they'll go a long way toward meeting that goal.

Physicians who are engaged and aligned are more successful in improving their own skill sets. We'll touch on this later in the book when we discuss the steps physicians can take to prevent and treat their own burnout. Physicians are more motivated than they've ever been before to make these tactics work. We all are.

You may have heard the adage "When the student is ready, the teacher appears." I believe a similar statement could be "When the environment is ready, the tactics can be more easily executed." That time is here.

Quint

INTRODUCTION

D*ecember 1, 2014, 7:00 p.m.*
I'm sitting in a patient care room at Doctors Hospital in Sarasota, Florida. I'm alone with my sister, Susan, my only sibling, seven years older than me, who passed away just minutes earlier. As I sit here with my sister, I make a commitment to her: Now that she is gone, I will take care of our mother and father. I don't realize that my father will pass away just two months from now. All I know as I sit here alone in a room with the sister I love, saying goodbye, is that her entire illness and particularly the hours before her death are flashing before me—and the calming presence of Dr. Pamela Hodul is there the whole time.

When Susan took her last breath, her husband, Jerry, was on her left side. Ruth Ann and Frank Miller, the dear friends who were with her from the beginning, were in the room. Pam Beitlich, a nurse at Sarasota Memorial Hospital who also works with Studer Group®, was there in the room, stunned because she had just seen Susan a day earlier and she seemed to be doing so much better. (In fact, they had been talking about going home.) I was there, next to her right hip. There, also next to her on the right side, holding her hand, was Dr. Hodul.

Dr. Hodul isn't on the medical staff at Doctors Hospital in Sarasota. She's a surgeon at Moffitt Cancer Center in Tampa, Florida. After I had texted her to say that things were bad, she'd gotten in her car and driven to Sarasota. She'd walked into the room and became completely intent on trying to save my sister's life. After asking the nurse and others a number of questions, it became apparent she couldn't do that. She took me out in the hall and said that Susan could not be saved. She went back in and she held Susan's hand, and Susan passed away.

On December 18, I heard from Dr. Hodul again. She had texted me a message, just saying that she knew it was Susan's birthday, and she knew that this would be a day that we were thinking about Susan and so was she. I don't think Dr. Hodul is the exception. I think she's the rule. She is a very, very dedicated physician, who sacrificed much of her own life in order to make a difference in the lives of other people.

I first met Dr. Hodul on September 13. On September 12, my sister had undergone an operation, a Whipple procedure, for pancreatic cancer. Frank and Ruth Miller were with her at the hospital, as was her husband, Jerry, while I stayed in Fort Meyers, FL, with my parents, Quinton and Shirley Studer. The next day, Jerry had to come home because of his own medical condition. It was then that we got word from Dr. Hodul that there were many complications. We had been expecting a stay in the ICU of about four to six days, followed by a 17-day hospital stay and then home care. Instead, a critical situation had developed. Mother looked at me and, without even a pause, said, "I want you there."

So I drove up there to Moffitt Cancer Center with my wife, Rishy, to be with my sister. We talked to Dr. Hodul, who I am sure was exhausted from the 13.5-hour surgery the day before on Susan. Later when I talked to Frank and Ruth Miller, who had been there after the surgery, they told me that Dr. Hodul had cried, totally exhausted. She said she had done everything she could because she had told Susan she was going to give it all she had.

Susan wasn't a great candidate for surgery. One could probably debate whether surgery should have been done. However, because of her extremely close relationship with our mother, she felt she had to try. My mother gave birth to my sister, Susan, during World War II. My father had gone into the Navy and was in the Pacific when Susan was born. In fact, Susan was three years old before my father even met her. For three years, it was just my sister and my mother, which created an unbelievable bond. Susan never could have children, so she and my mother became even closer. In fact, I used to joke that because they lived in the same condo development, my sister's big act of rebellion was that she moved across the street into a townhouse!

When my sister became ill, my mother had said to her, "I don't want you to die before me." This was not out of selfishness, but out of fear and sadness. This meant the only option my sister saw was to have this surgery after she was found to have pancreatic cancer. If she didn't have this surgery, she knew she would most likely die before my mother. So she begged and pleaded, and finally it was agreed upon that the surgery would happen.

From September all the way through December, there was always someone near Susan, either Frank and Ruth or myself. We had those "good days" that many of you who have had sick loved ones may be familiar with—those days that feel quite promising. Susan got transferred to the complex hospital in Sarasota. In fact, she was doing so well that we were setting up home healthcare for her, and she was going to go home on Tuesday, December 2. But you already know what happened on December 1.

We had some challenges throughout this process, but Susan's remarkable physicians were a constant. There were hospitalists in the ICU who were there constantly trying to make sure that Susan made it in her critical condition. There were pulmonologists, who seemed to be there constantly, trying to figure out what they could do to be helpful. And Dr. Hodul was the one we got to know the best. We saw her cry at times, when she was disappointed in what was going on. We saw her smile later when Susan was doing a little bit better. Yeah, I know that in healthcare you're not supposed to tie your emotions to other people, but how can you not? We all know physicians are people who care deeply about their patients.

Life can be really tough on physicians. One of my good friends, Dr. Ernie Deeds, is a case in point. As a young physician, he inherited a practice from a retiring physician named Dr. Guttman. When Ernie took over the practice, many of his patients were about 15-20 years older than him. Ultimately, he also retired from being a physician when he was 55 years old. One reason he gave me was that he had gone to three funerals in one week. He said he realized that the age of his patients meant that was pretty much what he'd always be doing and he just couldn't take it.

Dr. Hodul is another example. She's a young physician. She has spent most of her life getting her medical degree and completing her residency and then her fellowship so she could do the surgery that she loved. She knew that many of her patients had a bleak prognosis, so she has also chosen to do some procedures where the patients have a better chance for long-term survival.

I learned Dr. Hodul's schedule, and it was brutal. She would come in before 7:00 in the morning, many times even before 6:30, to see her hospitalized patients. Then she would either go on to do surgery on another patient—and these were long surgeries—or she would go to her outpatient clinic. She would stick around at night to make another round. She worked six days a week. On Sundays, she would periodically go to the computer just to check on how her patients were doing.

One time I asked Dr. Hodul about her social life, and she just sort of looked at me and said, "I really don't have time for that."

It hit me then, as it has before, the great price physicians pay to take care of us the way they do. Dr. Hodul and all the physicians who worked on Susan all those days and nights…what a sacrifice they make… And all physicians do this everywhere.

As I alluded to earlier, my father died not long after Susan, passing away on January 26, 2015. He was in Hope Hospice in Fort Myers, FL. The physician who was with him when he passed away had been an Emergency Department physician at one time. He told me he just couldn't do emergency medicine anymore, and that's why he was now a hospice physician—and he was a great one.

During all of these several months in hospitals, with my sister and then with my father, I talked to many physicians who are frustrated. They were frustrated at times because they wanted things done on the weekends that couldn't get done. They were frustrated that sometimes at 6:00 at night, certain things didn't run like they ran throughout the day.

They were also frustrated because of the new electronic medical record (EMR)—deep down they know it's going to be a good thing, but right now it's creating so much stress. They were upset because they're measured mostly on RVUs. Some of them are working harder than they ever worked in the past, and yet to other people looking at analytics and metrics, it looks like they're working less. I support analytics, metrics, EMRs, and RVUs. However, other things have to work well for those to work well, too.

I've been a big fan of physicians since early on in my career when I worked as the administrator on call and

I heard a doctor talking to a family about whether or not to resuscitate their father who was in the critical care unit. And now that I see all the massive changes physicians must endure, I admire them more than ever.

As I look back over the history of Studer Group, I question some things about myself and about what we have accomplished. We have done some great things, and there are some things I believe we could have done better—and one of the things I think we could have done better has to do with physicians. I'll come back to that, but first I will start with the positive.

We've been fortunate to win the Baldrige Award and a lot of other awards, but that's really not why we got into this work. We got into it to fulfill our mission statement, which is to make healthcare better for patients to receive care, for employees to work, and for physicians to practice medicine. When I look at the Baldrige Award and I look at our statistics, I can feel pretty good that we delivered on the first part of that promise, to make healthcare organizations better places for patients to receive care.

I feel really good about making healthcare a better environment in which employees can work. In the 1990s, I would see published healthcare to-do lists and I would notice that patients and employees were not in the top 10 of the to-do lists. I think we've done a very good job of helping put patients and employees much higher on those lists. In fact, I can't think of an organization that doesn't have patient experience as a top priority on their to-do list, or doesn't understand the importance of employee engagement.

Back in the early to mid-1990s, when I was working in a hospital, we needed a chief recruitment officer because we needed more nurses. We were paying nurses for 80 hours a week to work for 72 hours. We were spending a lot of money for agency nursing. And what we heard was that it was only going to get worse, because nurses were unhappy and disengaged. This was not because they wanted to be unhappy and disengaged, but because the quickly changing work environment created changes that were hard to adjust to quickly.

And so we made changes and improvements to make sure we recaptured the nurses. When I was at Holy Cross Hospital in Chicago and it won some awards, Tom Badal, an environmental services worker, was interviewed by a magazine. They asked Tom what the difference was between the hospital then and the hospital now. He said, "We used to worry about money and we lost it. Today we worry about people and we make it."

We knew if we didn't figure out a better way to make our organizations better places for all people to work, particularly nurses, we were going to be in big trouble. Today it's not like that. There are waiting lists for people wanting to go to nursing school. When somebody says they're going to be a nurse, they hear, "What a great profession." People are actually leaving other professions because they want to become nurses. Or they want to come into healthcare in some other capacity, like nurse practitioner, or physician assistant, or some other professions. But we don't hear that so much about physicians.

When I hold up the mirror and do my own self-inventory, I will admit that I've fallen short in making healthcare a better environment for physicians to practice medicine. We've written books on the subject of physician engagement. We have tactics that we know will work. But up until now I've never really figured out, to the level of expertise that I want at least, how to execute it all in the most effective possible way. And my career is going to be dedicated to finishing up what I hope we've started, which is creating better places for physicians to practice medicine.

As an industry, we've made a lot of leaps forward, and when I say "we," I mean you. We're more integrated than we've ever been before, which is a good thing. There is better technology, even though specific parts of it, like the electronic medical record, must get better. Many facilities are world class. There is more and more integration. We're figuring out how to create an aligned healthcare system. There is focus on how to manage population health, but if the physicians are not totally engaged—remember, engagement is the opposite of burnout—all of our efforts will fall short.

I'm on the board of a health system that has an exciting strategic plan. They have a nice geographic footprint. They have a lot of pieces in place, and people are working very hard. But, the physician engagement survey that recently came back was disappointing, as the results had gotten worse. My statement at the board meeting was "If we don't get physician engagement right, nothing else will matter."

That's where we are right now. How do we proactively engage physicians so they won't burn out? I'm optimistic we will, and I'm not blaming anyone. It's just that sometimes things happen. Life gets in the way. We have all these things hitting us at the same time. Healthcare is one of the most complex environments that exist. But there are bright spots out there. We see bright spots across the country. And that's what we do: As the Heath brothers, who wrote the book *Switch: How to Change Things When Change Is Hard*, would say, we find these bright spots and we learn from them.

What we've learned is many of the tactics we've written about are being implemented to some degree, but they can be very hard to execute consistently. Of course, there are also some tactics in this book that are new. If we implement these, and if we do a better job of executing the ones we already knew about, we will recapture the hearts and minds of physicians, just as we have done with other people in the healthcare profession.

As an industry, healthcare has accomplished remarkable things, and more remarkable things will be done in the future. I have no doubt. Physicians and health systems working together was always meant to be.

The title of this book is *Healing Physician Burnout* because there's every indication that burnout is here and it's a big challenge. But the most important part of the title is the first word: *Healing*. Our physicians really can heal and they really can be even better than they've ever been before. The working title for a while was *Who Moved My Future?* We meant it to be a *Who Moved My Cheese?* for doctors. The future *has* been moved; there's no doubt about it. But let's not make the move a bad thing. Let's make the move a good thing.

Thank you for your dedication and desire to create that special place for physicians so they enjoy practicing medicine. When the recruitment and retention of physicians takes place today, the foundation to attract the physicians for the next generation and the generation after that is set in place. Physicians have great purpose, do worthwhile work, and make a difference.

I'm grateful to have known many great physicians in my life. Thank you for all you've done and all you continue to do every day.

Quint

PART ONE:

WHY *ARE* PHYSICIANS SO BURNED OUT, ANYWAY?

E ffective medical care begins with understanding. Likewise, when we set out to help physicians overcome the burnout that many are experiencing, we must first know *why* they are experiencing it. There are many reasons. Ask any group of physicians why they believe they're feeling exhausted, dissatisfied, discouraged, helpless, and/or hopeless and there are any number of replies.

For example, one may hear, "I work too hard for too little pay-off. These brutal hours and endless bills are draining the life out of me."

Or, "I went to medical school so I could help patients, not to be buried in an avalanche of paper work."

Or, "I can't help patients to the extent I want. Even if I had enough time to really talk to them—which I don't— all they want to do is tell me what they read online."

Or just, "Government funding. Enough said."

Yes, there are many complicated and intertwined factors that are plunging too many physicians into a state of depression and burnout: uncertainty created by the ever-changing landscape of healthcare, a lack of control over their future, highly stressful jobs, bureaucratic pressure that interferes with optimal care, time constraints that keep them from forming meaningful patient relationships, salary concerns, and the feeling of being stuck in a career they no longer enjoy.

Meanwhile, many physicians are being evaluated to the greatest extent on relative value units (RVUs) as a comparable service measure and are under a lot of pressure to perform. Yet according to research, many physicians are not receiving the feedback or coaching on how to meet these performance standards or metrics.

And while physicians' income *is* high compared to most professions (though not nearly as high as many believe), they're burdened with massive education debt on top of their mortgages and other expenses. These financial realities force most physicians to keep practicing medicine whether they want to or not. (It's not like physicians can drop out of the game and "find themselves" while backpacking across Europe.)

It's no surprise that, as Sandeep Jauhar, MD, PhD, wrote in a 2014 *Wall Street Journal* article, "American doctors are suffering from a collective malaise. We strove, made sacrifices—and for what? For many of us, the job has become only that—a job."[1]

Indeed, according to an editorial published in the *Journal of General Internal Medicine*, burnout rates range from 30-65 percent across specialties such as critical care (53 percent), primary care (50 percent), and ED physicians (52 percent).[2]

What is burnout, anyway? A simple definition could be expressed as the "progressive loss of idealism, energy, and purpose."[3]

Psychologist Christina Maslach codified burnout in the MBI (Maslach Burnout Inventory). This 22-item inventory is broken down into three dimensions: Emotional Exhaustion, Cynicism, and Ineffectiveness. It has been the validated tool and gold standard for measuring burnout since the 1970s. (To access the MBI, please visit http://www.mindgarden.com/117-maslach-burnout-inventory.)

Here's a brief description of these three dimensions:

- **Emotional Exhaustion.** This is the sense of being emotionally drained while working with other people and the dread that accompanies thoughts of having to go to work. Rather than being energized by one's job, one is exhausted by it. It's the loss of the "passion" that's so fundamental to providing excellent healthcare.

- **Cynicism.** This dimension may also be expressed as depersonalization, withdrawal, and compassion fatigue. In short, the burned out person becomes numb to the humanity of others. In medicine this manifests as the physician no longer regarding the patient as a unique individual with fears, needs, and hopes. The patient becomes another "number," or just another member of a disease group (diabetic, hypertensive, etc.). The heart becomes "hardened," and empathy is lost.

- **Ineffectiveness/Lack of Efficacy.** Essentially, one loses their desire to accomplish great goals and make the world a better place. This is very serious, as physicians (much like nurses, teachers, ministers, and counselors) by their nature want to serve. The burned out clinician, who started out with such idealism, really begins to doubt that their work has purpose and that they are able to make a difference.

What's more, Geneia's Physician Misery Index Survey revealed that "two-thirds (67 percent) of all surveyed doctors know a physician who is likely to stop practicing medicine in the next five years, as the result of physician burnout. This includes both younger and more experienced doctors."[4]

The real surprise is that numbers like these aren't bigger—faced with the changes and challenges physicians deal with every day, who *wouldn't* be burned out?

In Part 1 we will discuss some of these issues. As I sat down and tried to make sense of all the "burnout factors" that are found in my own and others' researched perceptions (and that I know firsthand from my work with physicians across the country), it made sense to divide them into five major "groupings." These are:

- The Healthcare Environment
- Practical Hurdles
- Psychological Challenges
- Training Challenges
- Organizational Structure Changes

Of course, not all of the issues fall neatly into their assigned category. There is a fair amount of crossover. After all, practical hurdles often lead to psychological challenges. Training needs and adjusting to new organization structures are clearly related. The disconnect obviously has psychological implications, too. You get the picture: The lines are blurred.

Also, each factor is addressed, and I'd like to add that burnout *isn't* happening only because doctors feel personally overwhelmed, stressed, neglected, and put-upon. This would imply a lot of self-interest on the part of physicians, and that's just not true. I've worked with hundreds of physicians and I know their great dedication and stamina and their concern with their patients' well-being more than with their own. I find much of their burnout is due to the perception that their most powerful driver—the ability to provide the best possible patient care—is being challenged.

As a research report produced by the Rand Corporation and sponsored by the American Medical Association noted:

"We found that, when physicians perceived themselves as providing high-quality care or their practices as facilitating their delivery of such care, they reported better professional satisfaction. Conversely, physicians described obstacles to providing high-quality care as major sources of professional dissatisfaction. These obstacles could originate within the practice (e.g., a practice leadership unsupportive of quality improvement ideas) or could be imposed by payers (e.g., payers that refused to cover necessary medical services)."[5]

Without a doubt, many of the barriers we'll cover in Part 1 of this book are seen by physicians as challenges to their goal of providing high-quality healthcare. This is deeply upsetting to them. It's up to all of us collaboratively, as leaders and physicians alike, to work together to knock down these barriers. We need to a) assist physicians to master the tools and techniques to alleviate the obstacles that can be alleviated, and b) help physicians shift their perceptions to focus on the good that they've

always done for their patients and will continue to do—
whatever the future holds.

CHAPTER ONE:

"BIG PICTURE" CHANGES THAT ARE DRIVING DAY-TO-DAY REALITIES (THE HEALTHCARE ENVIRONMENT)

T he Affordable Care Act (ACA) has forever altered America's healthcare industry. And no one has seen more change than physicians. Many physicians have moved from solo practices or small groupings to joining ever-larger practices and systems. Employment has moved from solo to a group LLC to often a large organization. All kinds of changes are upon physicians—from how they get paid (and how much) to how they make decisions about treatment to how they interact with patients to how they keep records.

Coping with these pressures and new ways of doing things is incredibly stressful. The logistical and psychological implications are huge. And in the eye of this storm, under tremendous pressure to standardize care and reduce the cost of care, physicians keep on keeping on—doing everything possible to deliver the best possible clinical outcomes and improve efficiency, while keeping patients and their families informed and well cared for. Physicians have always *wanted* to do these things (it's a cornerstone of their calling), but new regulations and the ever-looming threat of withheld reimbursement have created an unprecedented sense of alarm.

The purpose here is not to cover every nuance of the external environment, but to offer an overview of the high spots. While these will not be new to most readers, putting them together helps better explain why physicians are feeling as they are today. Here are just a few of the big, overarching trends that are shaking up the healthcare industry:

Healthcare funding has reached worrisome levels. According to CMS.gov, healthcare spending now consumes 17.4 percent of gross domestic product (GDP). In 2013 spending on healthcare was $2.9 trillion, which comes out to $9,255 per person.[1]

If healthcare spending keeps growing at this rate, it will consume GDP—a course that is not feasible.

Value-based purchasing increasingly ties reimbursement to clinical quality and patient experience outcomes. This is a major paradigm shift from "services delivered" to "outcomes performed," and it includes both public and private payers. Not only does this new reality ramp up the pressures physicians feel to perform, it's counter to their "rugged individualist" roots.

Note that "quality" and "patient experience" both factor into reimbursement. CMS's value-based purchasing formula is linked both to quality metrics like outcomes and process of care measures and results on patient surveys: HCAHPS (for hospitals) and CG CAHPS (for physician practices). (The good news is that plenty of research shows quality and perception of care are two sides of the same coin.)

If you'd like to learn more about the quality/experience connection, I invite you to read *The CG CAHPS Handbook: A Guide to Improve Patient Experience and Clinical Outcomes*, by Jeff Morris, MD, MBA, FACS; Barbara Hotko, RN, MPA; and Matthew Bates, MPH; and *The HCAHPS Handbook: Tactics to Improve Quality and the Patient Experience*, by Lyn Ketelsen, RN, MBA; Karen Cook, RN; and Bekki Kennedy.

A physician shortage is imminent. Lots of attention has been focused on the upcoming shortage of primary care physicians (and in many parts of the country this is already a problem). But specialists, too, are becoming an endangered species. According to an article in the *Journal of Clinical Oncology*, "an acute shortage of medical oncologists is projected in the U.S. by 2020." This same article also referenced a 2007 survey projecting that the visit capacity of oncologists rising 14 percent by 2020 would be dwarfed by the projected demand of 48 percent![2] In general, it's estimated that there will be a deficit of 200,000 physicians by the year 2025.[3] This is a deeply alarming number and one that calls for changes in how we as an industry deliver care as well as how we fund and encourage physician education and training.

Meanwhile, our aging population will need more and more care. This physician shortage becomes even more serious when we consider the strain that 75 million aging baby boomers will place on those few who remain. According to a *Hospitals & Health Networks* article by Paul Barr titled "The Boomer Challenge," "About 3 million baby boomers will hit retirement age every year for about the next 20, and will affect how caregivers and policymakers shape the healthcare system for decades to come."[4]

The volume and acuity of healthcare needs have increased dramatically in last 40 years. Look at the explosion of diagnostic tools (ultrasound, CT, MRI), medications, and surgeries (both invasive and non-invasive) we've seen in recent decades. None of this existed in the early 1970s! Largely as a result of these medical advancements, people are living longer and consuming more healthcare of an intrinsically more expensive nature. The exponential growth of the cost of funding all of this is not sustainable.

Patient expectations have changed. The public's expectations and demand for healthcare have grown exponentially in the last 40 years. It's easy to see why. Medicine has delivered high quality and sometimes miracle cures. A strong "consumerism" orientation and perhaps even an element of entitlement have developed.[5] With increasing copays and deductibles, consumer intensity in selection of care providers and in what is expected in terms of treatments and outcomes will continue to grow.

The Internet is a big part of this. Now that it's so easy for people to do online research, they may sometimes come to doctor visits with preconceived ideas about what their treatment should be. Also, in a larger sense, the Digital Age has created a marketplace that favors the consumer. If you don't like what one company is offering, you can quickly and easily purchase goods and services from a competitor. This has taken the adage "the customer is always right" to new levels—and people naturally bring that same attitude to their healthcare.

There is more transparency than ever before. Thanks to the public reporting on Hospital Compare and Physician Compare websites, consumers can see how health systems, group practices, and individual clinicians are performing on certain quality and patient perception of care metrics. And, of course, thanks to social media, patients and families can post their healthcare experiences—positive or negative—at any time.

While transparency can be a very good thing, it can lead to discomfort in physicians. For example, physicians and organizations may feel that transparency may not accurately reflect their performance.

Technology is changing rapidly. Changes and advancements in technology, including electronic medical records (EMRs), cause discomfort as new skills are learned and demonstrated. As technology changes, there are more and more diagnostic and treatment options for patients. While more options is theoretically a good thing, the stress of having to learn about them all, and factor them into already-complex decisions on patient care, can contribute to burnout.

CHAPTER TWO:

THE DIRECT IMPACT ON PHYSICIANS (PRACTICAL HURDLES)

These trends have very real and often very painful consequences for physicians. All the industry changes they must navigate, all the mandates they must live up to, all the regulations that dictate how they must treat patients have transformed the modern physician's workday into one that's virtually unrecognizable to their forbears.

"The 'alphabet soup' physicians are to master—CPT, ICD-9, ICD-10, EMR—and the 'brain-numbing' number of hurdles physicians must leap just to deliver care to the patient—are issues that were unimaginable when I started my career in private practice of internal medicine in 1979," says Dr. George Ford.

Let's explore a few of the hurdles today's physicians have to overcome.

Physicians currently feel overworked. The Physicians Foundation's 2014 Survey of American

Physicians found that more than 80 percent of doctors say they are "overextended or at full capacity."[1] Another study reports that nearly 40 percent of physicians work more than 60 hours per week compared with only 10.8 percent of U.S. workers.[2]

Ironically, very few physicians would recommend such an unhealthy, unsustainable lifestyle for their patients. Physicians are only human, and all humans need a certain amount of down time for their mental and emotional health. Like everyone else, physicians need and deserve time for a life outside of work.

Many physicians are sleep deprived, too. While the sleep-deprived resident has almost become a cliché, physicians at all stages of their careers get too little sleep. There are many reasons why. If a surgeon is on call and has to come in for an emergency surgery in the middle of the night, and then has other scheduled surgeries the next day, they will clearly be operating on too little sleep. With cell phones and other technology providing 24/7 access to physicians, plus the long hours they spend trying to manage the changes in their work day, no wonder physicians go to bed too late, or simply don't get good sleep.

Most Americans are sleep deprived, so it's not surprising that this includes physicians. But of course when someone's life is held in your hands, working while sleepy is a bigger deal than if you're, say, a seamstress who accidentally cuts a dress too short. Besides making mistakes more likely to occur, prolonged sleep deprivation almost inevitably results in burnout.

Physicians feel they spend too little time with patients... Physicians want to spend most of their time with patients. That's why they went into medicine in the first place. Yet for a variety of reasons, physicians find themselves forced into frustratingly short appointments. No wonder a Geneia survey of more than 400 full-time physicians found that 78 percent of them "feel rushed" during their time with patients.[3]

A satisfied physician is a physician who feels confident their patients are getting the best possible care. A physician who feels "rushed" may not have that confidence. In fact, the AMA-sponsored Rand Corporation report "Factors Affecting Physician Professional Satisfaction and Their Implications for Patient Care, Health Systems, and Health Policy" noted that "Physicians in multiple specialties and all practice models included in this study described having insufficient time to deliver what they perceived as high-quality patient care."[4]

...and too much time doing everything else. The Rand report continues: "At the same time, however, many physicians—especially those without large numbers of dedicated allied health professionals and support staff—described spending a significant amount of time performing tasks that did not truly require a physician's training and that 'crowd out' those that did. For example, such activities as filling out forms, typing and correcting automated transcriptions, dealing with multiple EHR order entry screens, and other 'secretarial' duties were reported as occupying a significant share of physicians' time."[5]

Insurance alone is incredibly time-consuming. Sandeep Jauhar writes in his *Wall Street Journal* article, "U.S. doctors spend almost an hour on average each day, and $83,000 a year—four times their Canadian counterparts—dealing with the paperwork of insurance companies. Their office staffs spend more than seven hours a day."[6]

Physicians everywhere complain about the bureaucratic hoops they're forced to jump through—not just because they're time-consuming but because they're seen as not benefiting patients. Consider the following excerpt from "Survey: Bureaucracy Crushing Texas Physicians" posted on the Texas Medical Association website:

"More than half of Texas physicians (58 percent) say next year's forced upgrade to the government's new billing and coding system, ICD-10, will 'create a severe administration problem.' That is because ICD-10 will require doctors to use 69,000 diagnostic codes—up from the current system's 13,500 codes. All physicians, hospitals, providers, and insurance companies must shift from ICD-9 to ICD-10 by Oct. 1, 2015, but only 8 percent of Texas physicians say the shift will 'improve diagnosis or quality of care.' Many doctors believe ICD-10, 20 years in the making, is a boondoggle of a system that will help only healthcare researchers."[7]

Technology changes/EMR implementation brings another set of time pressures. Another big factor contributing to burnout is the explosion of technology and rapid changes that are needed as we use it to make improvements in patient care. Consider that in 2008 electronic medical record implementation was utilized in about 13 percent of offices, yet had risen to 72 percent in 2012.[8] That's a big leap, and it has taken its toll. While the EMR will eventually make life easier for many, that fact does not take away from the learning curve as physicians work to adjust and acquire new skills to implement it.

The same article also points out, "...primary care physicians who are using EMR with a moderate number of functions report more stress and less job satisfaction than physicians with low numbers of EMR functions."[9]

It's not hard to see why. While many physicians agree that EMR will be a good thing in the long run, getting accustomed to them is far from easy. There have also been some operational obstacles with some systems. This is not unusual with new technology. However, the length of time it takes to enter data, deal with cumbersome interfaces, and so forth may often have a significant impact upon physician productivity. (Physician may spend a lot more hours working with fewer RVU credits.)

Finally, it's not just that EMR recordkeeping is hard to get used to. The technology itself has serious challenges. As the Rand report I've cited previously puts it, "Few other service industries are exposed to universal and substantial incentives to adopt such a specific, highly regulated form of technology, which has, as our findings suggest, not yet matured. The current state of EHR technology appears to significantly worsen professional satisfaction for many physicians—sometimes in ways that raise concerns about effects on patient care."[10]

CHAPTER THREE:

THE STRESS OF COPING WITH UNPREDICTABILITY AND CHANGE (PSYCHOLOGICAL CHALLENGES)

I f one wants to visualize how it feels to be a physician in an unpredictable environment, consider what it's like to experience a flight delay. (I chose this example because I feel most people reading this book can relate.) We get to the airport at a certain time, based on having been told when the flight will leave. Then suddenly, because of an external environment event like the weather, or an internal environment event like a mechanical issue or the need to wait for a flight crew to arrive, a delay is announced.

Now sometimes the delays don't really matter because we have nothing else planned. But other times a delay can have serious consequences.

I've flown often enough that I've seen people miss key transfers that would have taken them to Europe or maybe to a wedding, and I've seen the emotional challenge that results. In 2010, when the Citi BCS National Championship Football Game was being held in Pasadena, CA—it was the Texas Longhorns versus the Alabama Crimson Tide—I was in the Dallas airport, and there were long delays. I remember some of the college football fans getting so upset because they might not get to the game on time, and the emotions were very, very raw.

Another time I was traveling to New York to be on the *Morning Joe* show, and I got to Atlanta and things were running late. I ran through the airport and was just about to the door when the door closed. I was actually standing at the window, looking at the pilots and trying to signal to them that I needed to get on the plane. Actually, I felt a lot like that little boy looking at a puppy through the glass in a pet store. But, of course, once the door is locked, the plane has to go.

I, of course, shared my displeasure with the airline person at the counter, and sat down to stew a little bit. Then I realized that I had to rebook my flight if I was going to make it to New York. And since this was the terminal where everyone was flying to New York, I was probably going to have to rebook with the fellow that I had just showed my displeasure. So of course I had to go up and say, "You know, I might have overreacted a little bit back there."

So if the football fans and I got so upset over these late or missed flights, which are infrequent events, think what a physician's life is like when things like this happen too often. If a physician is working in a hospital setting, they normally arrive at a certain time. It depends on when the first OR case is, or when they need to be there for patient rounds, or whatever. And maybe the physician has to get it all done before the outpatient clinic they're running that afternoon. So when something happens to delay the expected schedule, the entire day gets shifted around. Everybody gets frustrated, upset, and anxious.

Let's say I'm a physician waiting for a test result that's supposed to be done at a certain time. And let's say it isn't done in time. Then I have a family who's extremely upset. When they're upset with healthcare, they're generally also upset with me personally. Or if I'm in an outpatient clinic and the patient comes in and has to wait for a long time, or there's a problem with their tests or treatment, the same thing happens. There's just a lot of confusion and stress.

For example, when my sister was being treated for pancreatic cancer (a story I shared in the Introduction to this book), she was told to fast on Friday because her physician was going to do a surgical procedure at noon. The procedure ended up happening at 8:30 that night, which meant she went through a whole day of fasting. They didn't get done till 10:30 p.m. Not only was this long delay discomforting to my sister and our family, I know it must have thrown the entire schedule off for that physician.

Of course, these things happen in healthcare. Some things can't be avoided. There may be an emergency or an accident, or even a series of traumas that create a domino effect of delays. We all understand that—but it still doesn't change the frustration that occurs when your schedule constantly gets shifted.

As I shared, I've made the analogy that being a physician is sort of like having to go to an airport five or six days a week. When you look at the airline data, that means that about 20 percent of the time you're going to have a delay or you're going to miss a flight. Emotionally, how would you handle that kind of life? Even if you're a very mature person, sometimes you are going to be frustrated when you constantly have to deal with these types of delays. After all, they not only impact your professional life but your personal life as well (every physician has most likely missed out on some important events and special moments with family and friends due to work delays and emergencies).

Now, on top of the daily stresses that are just part of the physician's life, they have to cope with all the massive shifts that are happening in healthcare. Of course, different physicians handle these changes in different ways.

All change is stressful. Yet while Person A may experience a particular change as deeply upsetting, Person B may experience the same change as exciting and stimulating. It depends on perception. The times we're living in aren't easy for most, but I believe it's best to accept change as it comes and focus on the constants that remain: our passion for the work, our commitment to providing great care, and our desire to make a difference. All the while we also need to understand that *acceptance* does not always mean *liking*.

That said, there are certain burnout factors that have a heavy psychological component for most physicians. Again, we will discuss them one at a time.

Physicians are experiencing a severe loss of control or the perception of loss of control. I bring this one up first for a reason. All the changes we've discussed so far (and all the ones still to be discussed) have taken away the physician's decision making over many aspects of their professional life—from income to scheduling to referral decisions to treatment plans. And it's probably not surprising that the Rand/AMA report I've already cited states, "Greater physician autonomy and greater control over the pace and content of clinical work were both associated with better professional satisfaction."[1]

In his book *Stop Physician Burnout: What to Do When Working Harder Isn't Working,* Dike Drummond, MD, says that in their medical training physicians are subject to five flavors of conditioning: *Workaholic, Superhero, Emotion-free, Lone Ranger,* and *Perfectionist.* His point is that this programming sets physicians up for future burnout.[2] I agree. I also feel that it instills a deep need in physicians to work in the way that they feel is right for themselves and their patients—which, in turn, makes it difficult when certain decisions are taken out of their hands.

In my view, physicians' current frustration is not because they crave authority. It's more that they crave respect for their ability to make decisions. Physicians are dismayed if they feel they are being pushed to work in a way that is not comfortable for them, not in the best interests of their patients, not according to their training and even their gut feeling about what is right.

There has been too much change, too fast. Few of us love change, especially when we are not the ones leading the change. This is not a "physician thing" but a "human thing." And when too many big changes happen in rapid succession, it's easy to feel overwhelmed and even panicky (like Lucy trying to keep up with the conveyor belt in the famous "chocolate factory" episode).

Consider the phases of change all people in all fields go through during their lives and careers.

Phase One: Unconsciously Unskilled— During this phase, we are new to a role, process, or skill. We don't know what we don't know because it is still too new.

Phase Two: Consciously Unskilled—In this phase, we consciously know what we don't know. We've identified a gap between our current skill set and where we need to be to become successful. This is called "creative tension."

Phase Three: Consciously Skilled—Here we have the skill set, but we still need reminders or checklists to fully execute. We are likely still unsettled, but we understand the need for change and have begun embracing it.

Phase Four: Unconsciously Skilled—It's in this phase that we can complete tasks without reminders. They have become second nature and we can't imagine doing it any other way.[3]

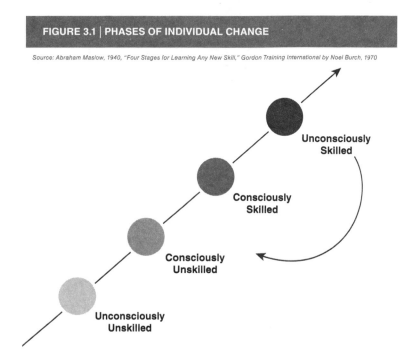

FIGURE 3.1 | PHASES OF INDIVIDUAL CHANGE

Source: Abraham Maslow, 1940, "Four Stages for Learning Any New Skill," Gordon Training International by Noel Burch, 1970

Imagine, then, how physicians who have been practicing for a while must feel when so much starts to shift, and more and more responsibility is piled on them. Through education, frequent repetition, and development, physicians have become "unconsciously skilled"—meaning they are able to work with a great ability to multi-task. Physicians are high performers. Now, suddenly, they are expected to master skills, some of which may not come naturally like their clinical learnings. They've gone backward to "consciously unskilled"—and that doesn't feel very good.

The physician may not say, "This is why I am feeling like I am feeling." They most likely will instead use something else as a reason for their discomfort. What we have found from working with hundreds of high-performing people is that this sense of going backward is underestimated, so sometimes individuals push back on change, and in reality it is not the change they are pushing back on, but instead the feeling of going backward when they want to maintain a high performance level.

If this is not understood by leaders, physicians may not get the needed time to adjust to a new skill so they can move themselves back up to an "unconsciously skilled" level. This does not mean that we may not coach them in new skills, techniques, and procedures. What it does mean is that we need to have great empathy for what physicians are going through. We can take that empathy and perhaps adjust RVUs for a while as they adjust to the change, or look at different ways to measure physician performance. We might take a look at what can be fixed around them to give the physician more time. These are the things that help a physician adjust.

Physicians face downward pressure in compensation, coupled with heavy debt. Not only are physicians being asked to relinquish control over their own lives and to change many things about the way they're used to working, they're now hearing, "Oh, yes, now we want you to do this for less money, or at least the same money."

In his *Wall Street Journal* article, Sandeep Jauhar writes, "In 1970, the average inflation-adjusted income of general practitioners was $185,000. In 2010, it was

$161,000, despite a near doubling of the number of patients that doctors see a day."[4]

Of course, by the standards of the rest of the world this is pretty good money. And certain specialties make better still. Even so, there is definitely a downward pressure on physician incomes, and some physicians may find themselves no longer making the salary they are accustomed to making.

This change in income represents a massive shift in the "social contract" physicians have always operated under. This creates a feeling that the rules have been changed in the middle of the game. When rules are changed during a game, most likely people will feel "this is not fair."

Plus, medical school is not getting any cheaper. According to the Association of American Medical Colleges (AAMC), "In 2013–2014, annual tuition and fees at public medical schools averaged approximately $31,783 for state residents and $55,294 for non-residents. At private schools, tuition and fees averaged $52,093 for residents and $50,476 for non-resident students. These figures do not include health insurance, housing, or living expenses."[5]

The same source notes that "in 2013, the median debt for graduating students was $175,000."[6] And while it's true that in most cases this is a sound investment, the emotional weight of owing this much money on top of ever-rising living expenses cannot be underestimated. Once physicians take on a mortgage (often a sizeable one) and possibly marry and have children, the financial burden can feel crushing. It can create the feeling of being a financial hostage.

In her Medscape.com article *Physician Burnout: It Just Keeps Getting Worse,* Carol Peckham discussed the results of Medscape's Physician Lifestyle Report 2015. She wrote, "In this year's Medscape survey, physicians were asked whether they had sufficient savings and/or an unacceptable degree of debt for the stage in life. Internists, family physicians, and intensivists, who are among the most burned-out physicians, were also among the least confident in their financial status."[7]

Physicians face a growing sense of "disconnection" from patients and community. Medicine has become more depersonalized. The reasons why are evident: more bureaucracy, more technology, less time to spend with patients, and increasing frustration (and even resentment) on both ends of the stethoscope. A sense of intellectual and emotional detachment between patient and physician has become the norm.

Certain physicians—for example, critical care and ER docs—most of the time don't have long-term relationships with patients. Now, the problem is spreading. The wise, kindly, hardworking doctor who patients trusted, admired, and counted on throughout life now feels like a relic from the 1950s or even longer ago. The system makes it so hard for this kind of bond to exist now—and the loss is as profound for physicians as it is for patients.

I've had physicians tell me they used to regularly receive cards from patients but that now they almost never do. Even today with the ease of communication created by email and text, good notes can get lost in the barrage of other activities.

All physicians of every age and in every field want and need to feel appreciated by and connected to their patients. It's what keeps them going even in the midst of tough financial and practical challenges. Take that connection away, and burnout is almost inevitable.

On top of everything else, physicians must cope with the inherent stress of practicing medicine. Even in the best of circumstances, practicing medicine is a very tough, very demanding job. I've read various articles on the subject of job stress, and in most of them physicians are listed right in line with professions like military, law enforcement, and firefighting. It's no coincidence that all these careers involve dealing with death, danger, and lots of raw emotion on a daily basis.

If you're a surgeon, it's your job to literally slice into a person's brain or heart or some other fragile and vital body part. If you're a family physician, it falls to you to (for example) prescribe the medication that's most likely to help and least likely to cause harm. Physicians bring people face to face with their own mortality. Physicians must tell parents the news that their child has died. Even on a "good" day, physicians deal with patients who are sick or in pain or anxious or worried. Very few people in other fields deal with such consistent pressure.

To me, one of the most powerful images showing what it means to be a physician was a photo that went viral. It showed an ER doctor hunched over, grief-stricken, by a concrete wall in a rainy parking lot at night.

He had just lost a 19-year-old patient. The person who posted the photo on Reddit.com has apparently since removed it, but someone sent me a link to a news story that reported what he had written:

"The man pictured was unable to save one of his patients. Though this is a common occurrence in our field of work, the patients we lose are typically old, sick, or some combination of the two. The patient that died was 19 years old, and for him, it was one of those calls we get sometimes that just hits you," wrote redditor Nick-Moore911. "Within a few minutes, the doctor stepped back inside, holding his head high again."[8]

CHAPTER FOUR:

PHYSICIANS ARE STRUGGLING WITH A LACK OF NEEDED SKILLS (TRAINING CHALLENGES)

I t's no secret that there's a general challenge in education around the skills being taught and the skills students will need to know after they graduate. School systems at every level are struggling to figure out how to prepare young people for a workplace forever changed by technology and globalization. Today's employees, and definitely tomorrow's, should be able to collaborate, innovate, and problem solve. These skills can't always be learned sitting in a classroom, listening to lectures, and memorizing facts—and that's why schools are working so hard to reinvent themselves.

Well, medical schools have a similar challenge. As a recent NPR article by Julie Rovner notes, "Most medical schools still operate under a model pioneered in the early 1900s by an educator named Abraham Flexner." The article goes on to explain that "Flexner's model is known as 'two plus two.' Students spend their first two years in the classroom memorizing facts. In the last two years, med students shadow doctors in hospitals and clinics."[1]

Another gap is that nurses and doctors are not trained together. This hampers their ability to form strong teamwork skills early on, which could in turn have a positive impact on burnout.

Just as the global business workplace is changing rapidly (and some might say relentlessly), so is the healthcare system. What worked yesterday doesn't work so well today and will work even less well tomorrow. Leaders in healthcare education know this and are working diligently on solutions.

In fact, the NPR article I just quoted is all about how medical schools are "rebooting" to help physicians develop the skills they'll need to thrive in a dramatically changing industry. Specifically they're working to help students develop skills like teamwork, communication, problem solving, and resiliency.

To help make the needed changes, the AMA recently gave $1 million to each of 11 medical schools through an initiative called "Accelerating Change in Medical Education." According to the AMA website, one recipient, Mayo Medical School, "aims to create a new educational model to prepare students to practice and lead within patient-centered, community-oriented, science-driven collaborative care teams that deliver high-value care."[2]

That said, here are a few of the training-related issues many of today's physicians face:

Many physicians need additional skills today beyond great clinical expertise. A recent *Wall Street Journal* article by Melinda Beck explains: "'The fund of medical knowledge is now growing and changing too fast for humans to keep up with, and the facts you memorize today might not be relevant five years from now,' says NYU's Dr. Triola. Instead, what's important is teaching 'information-seeking behavior,' he says, such as what sources to trust and how to avoid information overload.'"[3]

The additional skills needed today include: the ability to navigate electronic medical records, to consult a patient's economic "big picture" when ordering tests, to work in teams with other professionals who aren't doctors (and to be okay with not always knowing the answer), to communicate clearly, to engage patients as partners, and to know LEAN (process improvement) and cost reduction strategies.

Having to practice medicine in a time when many things are becoming obsolete is incredibly stressful. Not only is it hard to do a great job, but there's an emotional toll associated with the feeling that the change is passing one by.

However, change is constant. In John Kotter's book *A Sense of Urgency*, he discusses the difference between episodic change and continuous change. In healthcare, many of us have lived in an episodic change environment for many years. For example, codes were written and stayed that way for a long time. A budget was in place and it lasted 12 months. Capital improvements were approved and set for 12 months. A survey was done and everyone knew the time it was going to happen.

Now, however, all of a sudden, a budget is based only on volume, acuity, and payer mix. If any of these change, the whole entire budget changes. Something that was approved as a capital requirement is now taken off of the books when the health system receives a financial hit. The fact that the surveyors can come at any time, unannounced, creates additional pressure. Now with CG CAHPS/HCAHPS, instead of saying, "Did someone explain the side effects of medications?" it is, "Did they always explain the side effects of medications?"

What's happening in healthcare is that it has moved from an episodic change culture to a continuous change culture. As John Kotter states, there is nothing more difficult for an industry, and it can implode a culture. It is like going from knowing you're going to make Thanksgiving dinner one day a year to being prepared to make Thanksgiving dinner every day of the year.

We will eventually get there and adjust, but it means a huge overhaul of the processes and systems currently in place. Physicians and everyone else in healthcare are living and experiencing these changes now. Yet a physician can sometimes see the transition as more difficult because the decisions they make may save lives. This is a lot of pressure.

Physicians are rugged individualists who must learn to work in teams. It's no secret that physicians tend to have a certain personality type. Remember Dr. Dike Drummond's five flavors of physician conditioning? (To refresh your memory, they are *Workaholic, Superhero, Emotion-free, Lone Ranger,* and *Perfectionist.*) At least two of them—Lone Ranger and Superhero—underscore the fact that physicians are trained to be strong, capable, and independent. Like many characteristics, even good ones have unintended consequences.

Medicine has become much more of a team sport. Physicians are being asked to work collaboratively with other care providers like nurses, nurse practitioners, physician assistants, and pharmacists. Their training has been focused on technical skills—yet now physicians are expected not just to coordinate with but also to coach and inspire other team members. However, their performance may still be based on a productivity model.

Many new voices have become involved in treating patients. With the rise of the Internet, people have more and more information. Some of this information is correct; a lot of it is not correct.

Over the past couple of decades, it has gotten much easier for patients to research conditions and treatment options—including natural remedies—and to show up for appointments armed with specific ideas about what they need and want. Sometimes they're on the same page with the physician, sometimes not. Sometimes they're trusting, other times deeply skeptical. Regardless, treating today's patient is more complex than ever.

It's not surprising that this development is tough on physicians. Doing so requires more time. If physicians are not trained on how to communicate with respect and empathy, they can alienate patients.

Physicians who don't have superb communication skills can become frustrated as patients are not as compliant as they were years ago. This can negatively affect outcomes. All of this adds to the stress physicians are already under.

Patients have longer life spans, and their issues tend to be more complex. As patients live longer, they often develop more and more health challenges. It's not uncommon for a patient to have three or four or even five chronic conditions at the same time—say, obesity, congestive heart failure, hypertension, diabetes, and asthma. These patients tend to be on many different medications and are "prescribed" a certain type of diet and exercise plan. In other words, their care plan is extremely complex and demanding.

Now it is very unlikely that even the most well-meaning patient with a string of chronic conditions will follow their plan to the letter. Logistically, it's hard to remember to take four or five prescriptions every day without fail (and that's not even accounting for patients who quit because of unpleasant side effects). And let's be real: The patient probably isn't exercising three to five times a week either, and they're probably ordering the burger and milkshake more often than they do the baked fish and broccoli.

In other words, the patient is noncompliant. Add in the fact that physicians have less time with patients, which affects their ability to build a strong relationship and exert a positive influence, and it's easy to see why this is so frustrating. For one thing, physicians care about their patients and really want them to do better. But also, if physicians are being reimbursed based on outcomes, noncompliant patients can impact the bank account. It's stressful in the same way that middle management is stressful: You're responsible for the behavior of those over whom you have no real authority.

Patients expect miracles. Many of the treatment options we have now didn't exist years ago. While these recent advances have been great for many patients, they've also created incredibly high expectations across the board. Patients believe their doctors can solve any medical issue and save any patient—and obviously this is not true.

As a result, physicians sometimes have to deliver tough news that people don't want to hear. This in itself can be exhausting.

Physician attitudes toward work-life balance are changing. This may bring its own set of challenges. Consider the following passage from "Wanting It All: A New Generation of Doctors Places Higher Value on Work-Life Balance," an AAMC.org article by Eve Glicksman:

"The standard used to be 'more work, less life,' said Abdulla Ghori, MD, chair of graduate medical education and director of the Pediatric Residency Program at MetroHealth System in Cleveland, about previous generations of physicians. Residents work hard at the hospital, he said, but often do not have the energy or commitment to read more about a patient's condition once they go home. 'Just knowing the minimum required is not a healthy trend in the quality of physicians we train. That's where work-life balance becomes a problem.'"[4]

All of these issues exacerbate physician burnout. The good news is that medical schools are definitely aware of the growing burnout problem and are taking steps to address it at the student level. Remember the AMA's million-dollar grant to the Mayo Clinic? One of the concerns it will address is burnout.

The AMA website says, "As physician well-being impacts patient outcomes and access to care, Mayo and others are also developing tools and curriculum to enhance student well-being and resiliency. Mayo is testing the functionality of a Medical Student Well-Being Index, which allows self-assessment of distress and immediate access to local and national resources. The school has also created wellness learning modules and implemented a required curriculum focused on wellness and resiliency with facilitated small group modules."[5]

This out-of-the-box thinking addresses physician burnout as well as overall physician well-being. It is surely a step in the right direction.

CHAPTER FIVE:

PHYSICIANS NEED TO ADAPT TO NEW EMPLOYMENT REALITIES (ORGANIZATIONAL STRUCTURE CHANGES)

I t's getting more and more common for physicians to be employed by health systems and other large organizations. In fact, a recent Mayo Clinic *Proceedings* article titled "Impact of Organizational Leadership on Physician Burnout and Satisfaction" said, "Studies suggest that approximately 75 percent of U.S. physicians are now employed by hospitals, academic medical centers, health maintenance organizations, and large practice groups. This represents a profound structural change from the solo practitioner and small group practice models in which most physicians previously functioned."[1]

Whether it's due to direct employment or some other form of integration, the "ties that bind" health systems and physicians are tightening. I like the marriage analogy. It's as if the eternal reimbursement environment is pushing health systems and physicians into matrimony. Health systems need to make sure they're the kind of organization physicians will *want* to become part of. Like any other relationship, strong health system/physician partnerships take communication, hard work, and compromise on both sides.

Many organizations are doing great things in physician integration and engagement. Yet even in the best of circumstances, there is intense pressure around how the organization runs contrasted with how physicians work. The intense pressure of a new employment structure naturally heightens the stress so many physicians are already under for other reasons. This is not easy for other healthcare leaders either—but the good news is that there are solutions.

We're getting ready to explore a few of the most notable burnout factors below, but first I want to point out that many of them connect to the "loss of control" physicians are already feeling. Physicians deeply value autonomy, and when they are required to follow the rules and guidelines of the organization they're affiliated with, they lose some of that autonomy. Even when they know it's for the greater good (for instance, financial stability and efficiency of care), it's not easy for physicians to cope with the loss of control.

That said, here are a few issues connected to the health system/physician relationship that over time can lead to burnout:

Physicians desire development beyond clinical expertise. Once physicians have graduated from medical school, they may be viewed as a "finished product." This is a problem that will impact their entire career with the health system.

While physicians have always desired to keep their clinical knowledge and skills up to date, no wonder there is creative tension between physicians and other health system leaders and staff members! Now they are also expected to acquire many enhanced skills from technology to process improvement, work flow, clinical redesign, community, teamwork, and leadership. The good news is that health systems are increasing these development opportunities for physicians, especially in leadership, more and more.

Of course, such development opportunities are not always available, and if they are, time to meet and learn leadership skills is in short supply. Physicians are appreciative and health systems perform better when physicians have access to robust professional development. Take time to learn what the physician needs and provide them with all the tools they need to thrive—and to provide the best possible care to patients, which is always their top priority.

Consistently high quality operations are a must. Above all else, physicians care about patient outcomes. Physicians need to know their patients are well taken care of, and if they don't feel this is happening, they're going to be anxious and stressed. Providing consistent and exceptional quality care—meaning quality care that occurs with every patient, every department, every time—remains elusive for many.

The move to continuous change, transparency, and the need to cut costs while improving consistency can be difficult for health systems. All health systems can provide excellent operations from time to time, but too often cannot be sustained 24/7, 365 days a year. This is incredibly frustrating to physicians and may become a barrier to getting feedback from them. Physicians think, *Well, I've told them before what they need to fix and they still can't fix it, or they do but it doesn't stay fixed. Why bother?*

Physicians want to receive consistent performance feedback. Between 30 and 50 percent of physicians report they do not receive adequate or meaningful feedback on performance.[2] This shortfall creates many problems. When physicians don't know where they need to improve, it stands to reason that they can't, and won't, do so. This can negatively impact patient care but it can also impact physician compensation.

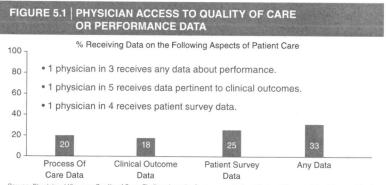

FIGURE 5.1 | PHYSICIAN ACCESS TO QUALITY OF CARE OR PERFORMANCE DATA

% Receiving Data on the Following Aspects of Patient Care

• 1 physician in 3 receives any data about performance.
• 1 physician in 5 receives data pertinent to clinical outcomes.
• 1 physician in 4 receives patient survey data.

Process Of Care Data	Clinical Outcome Data	Patient Survey Data	Any Data
20	18	25	33

Source: Physicians' Views on Quality of Care: Findings from the Commonwealth Fund National Survey of Physicians and Quality of Care; Anne-Marie J. Audet, Michelle M Doty, Jamil Shamsdin, & Stephen C. Schoenbaum; May 2005

Physicians benefit (as does the organization) from clearly defined and very specific goals that are aligned with the organization's larger goals. Physicians also need relevant, objective metrics built into their feedback. Physicians like facts and figures, and it will be a struggle to engage them in collaborative dialogue if one can't cite "the numbers."

Ultimately, physicians are just like everyone else in that they a) appreciate clarity around whether or not they are meeting expectations, and b) know exactly what needs to happen in order for them to meet expectations. Vagueness in either area results in uncertainty, which results in stress. Clarity and directness dissolve stress.

Studer Group® has created the Provider Feedback System[SM] to help create this kind of clarity. It collects and summarizes results in a way that aligns physician goals with the health system goals and shows physician performance over time. It actually shows individual provider movement from baseline. Ultimately, the idea is to encourage collaboration and to make sure organizations and physicians work together in a partnership that's good for all stakeholders—including, of course, the patients.

Physicians want to understand and be a part of the change process. Many health systems are making positive changes. Healthcare systems must now reinvent themselves—today's external healthcare environment demands it. Of course this reinventing is going on while they are moving forward, which is similar to enhancing the car's performance while you are driving.

There are no pit stops for healthcare leaders and organizations.

Physicians want to be part of the solution—there is no way the needed transformation will happen without their input and, most important, their support. Physicians are loaded with good ideas. The challenge is they often have little to no face time to discuss them.

Physician leader selection must be razor sharp. This is one of the issues pinpointed in the Mayo Clinic *Proceedings* article I mentioned earlier. The abstract states: "The leadership qualities of physician supervisors appear to impact the well-being and satisfaction of individual physicians working in healthcare organizations. These findings have important implications for the selection and training of physician leaders and provide new insights into organizational factors that affect physician well-being."[3]

A *HealthLeaders Media* article about this study— "Physician Burnout Heavily Influenced by Leadership Behaviors," by Alexandra Wilson Pecci—points out that physician leaders are often selected because they're accomplished clinicians or experts, *not* because they have great leadership skills.

Pecci quotes Tait Shanafelt, MD, professor of medicine at Mayo Clinic and first author of the study as saying, "'Those [clinical] qualities, while certainly admirable, may or may not set them up to succeed as a leader.'" Pecci then goes on to add, "Rather, other qualities, such as being open to new ideas, consensus building, and bringing together diverse opinions, are ones that make good leaders who can bring about change."

In the same article Pecci adds, "Shanafelt says the specific leadership behaviors he and his team evaluated could be boiled down into how well the supervisors informed, engaged, and empowered those that they led. He points out that all of the leadership behaviors measured were actionable, ones that can be learned or developed."[4]

It's so important for healthcare organizations to select physicians who have the right raw materials (and the right attitude) to be great leaders and to provide them well with the specific skills they'll need to educate and inspire others. If poor physician leadership contributes to burnout, it stands to reason that great physician leadership may prevent and even alleviate it.

Ochsner Health System in New Orleans has taken bold steps to work with their physician leaders to promote physician engagement and alignment across the system. After a thorough assessment and review of physician engagement results, deliberate strategies to promote engagement and alignment were introduced. Over 120 physician leaders received training on key leadership skills including physician rounding; effective use of stoplight reports; focus, fix, and follow-up; as well as reward and recognition. They also put into place an accountability mechanism to create and ensure alignment across the system.

Communication between physicians and staff is getting harder. Every physician knows this scenario: A nurse calls during the course of a busy day to talk about a patient. As the conversation unfolds, the physician asks a question. The nurse says, "Hold on, Doctor, let me pull up the information on the computer." This may seem like a small annoyance, but when it happens over and over, it can waste a lot of time.

Here's another example. Each physician likes to do things differently, and if staff members don't know these preferences—say, how each physician likes to round or how they prefer to be contacted—it leads to communication breakdowns and process inefficiencies. Everyone's day is disrupted (physicians' and staff members' alike). When you're seeking to help someone feel connected to your organization, it's smart to make an effort to learn how they do their best work—and to accommodate their preferences.

None of these examples—what they really are is bad interaction habits—are deal breakers on their own. But add them all together, and they become a huge stumbling block. Organizations want to create the right kinds of habits and standardize physician/staff interactions so that quality, efficiency, and safety are assured. This, however, takes time. In *Good to Great,* Jim Collins writes that moving to great is a complex task that happens over an 8- to 12-year timeframe.

All of the challenges we've discussed connect to the larger issue of physician engagement (which, as I've already noted, is the opposite of physician burnout). And we can talk about physician engagement all day long, but the reality is, people will naturally be more engaged when they are able to be highly productive. We all want to provide physicians with well-run organizations that support them, allow them to do their best work, and consistently deliver the highest quality patient care possible. This, more than any other perk or benefit or intervention, will decrease the likelihood of physician burnout.

PART TWO:

WHY PHYSICIAN BURNOUT MATTERS TO HEALTH SYSTEMS

CHAPTER SIX:

NINE WAYS BURNOUT HURTS PATIENTS AND ORGANIZATIONAL PERFORMANCE

S o much of the change needed in healthcare—
improving quality while reducing costs—depends on
physicians. We hear and read that the pressure on physicians is great. Physicians need to be fully aligned with
the goals of the organization, fully engaged in the clinical and leadership tactics proven to get results, and fully
present in their interactions with patients. For all of this
to happen, physicians have to be at the top of their game,
physically, mentally, and emotionally. And as we'll discuss
in Part 3, burnout impacts every area of a physician's
well-being: body, mind, and spirit.

All this means it's crucial that organizations laser-fo-
cus on the problem of physician burnout. This doesn't
mean merely being "aware of it" or "concerned about
it." Organizations need to be *absolutely committed* to recognizing, alleviating, and preventing physician burnout.
Actually, they need to make it a burning platform and

treat it with the sense of urgency it deserves. Healthcare leaders get these points. The difficult challenge is how to do it with so many other pressing issues facing healthcare providers.

From a purely financial standpoint, preventing and treating physician burnout just makes good sense. A healthcare system's largest producer of revenue is the medical staff. Most professions make a special point to take great care of their revenue producers. Healthcare can be no different. In healthcare, physicians are way more than the people who create the documentation for billing. They are the lifeblood of healthcare; they are the healers.

Health systems have always worked diligently to create that great place for physicians to practice medicine. Not too long ago, a hospital may have been called "the physicians' workshop." Healthcare leaders continue to strive to provide physicians with up-to-date technology, excellent facilities, and a well-trained staff. We know when any one of these three is not working well, it causes frustration for all in healthcare.

The challenge now is that so much needs to happen in addition to what might be called "the basics." Changes in the external environment in the areas of reimbursement and technology beyond patient diagnosis have created new structures health systems must work within, and many of these are in the early stages of operations. In addition, the implementation of electronic medical records (EMRs) and a focus on quick patient access to care have led to an environment of continuous change. (We know from John Kotter that moving from a state of episodic change to one of continuous change is stressful.) Even the most well-run organizations are challenged by multiple occurrences at the same time.

The good news is that a genuine sense of purpose—making patients' lives better—fuels our entire industry and underlies every decision that is made. This truth, more than anything else, makes a renewed focus on physician well-being a natural priority for healthcare organizations. Why? *Because the better we make doctors' lives, the better we make patients' lives.*

Health systems have always cared about physician burnout and many have taken steps to alleviate it in the past. For example, they've adopted tactics to get physicians aligned and engaged. But now that more and more physicians are employees (or at least becoming more tied to health systems through, say, accountable care organization arrangements), leaders are feeling the need to take bolder action.

As mentioned earlier, the external healthcare environment has now evolved to a place where leaders and physicians are more or less on the same page. Leaders want physicians to be aligned and engaged, and physicians want that too. The common understanding of the goal is there. It is the road to get there that is bumpy—and it can feel like we're driving a nitroglycerin truck over the rough spots. However, what needs to happen can't happen when so many physicians are struggling with burnout. Treatment for burnout must be addressed for physicians to be fully aligned and engaged—and the good news is that many times, the same tactics help accomplish all three goals.

Let's take a look at some specific ways physician burnout can harm patients and organizational performance:

Physician burnout threatens patient safety. This is probably the most pressing reason to deal with burnout. Common sense tells us that a burned out physician is less attentive to patient well-being and is thus more likely to make mistakes. Research backs up this supposition. For example, in a 2010 article in the *Annals of Surgery*, Shanafelt and his colleagues reported that 8.9 percent of 7,905 American surgeons reported having committed a major medical error in the preceding three months. Many of these physicians manifested burnout.[1]

Another study, this one focused on medical residents at the Mayo Clinic, found 34 percent of residents had a "major medical error," and this was correlated with burnout.[2]

No doubt these studies represent only the tip of the iceberg and do not include the many "near misses" that may occur. In that regard, healthcare compares to nuclear power plants or other organizations that do complex, high-stakes work.

Burnout can hurt clinical outcomes. An article published in *Health Care Management Review*, written by Jonathon R. B. Halbesleben and Cheryl Rathert, reported the findings of a study done on 178 physicians and their patients. Its findings suggested that "the depersonalization dimension of physician burnout was associated with patient outcomes of lower satisfaction and longer post-discharge recovery time."[3]

This is interesting on two counts. Obviously, the "longer recovery time" cited in the study means that patients are staying for longer than they need to. But also, we know from our experience coaching organizations that patient perception of care and clinical quality go hand in hand. When one improves, so does the other. When one goes down, so does the other.

Another study, one that summarized evidence from 55 studies, supports this connection between perception of care and clinical quality. The study, published in *BMJ Open* and written by Cathal Doyle and colleagues, found "consistent positive associations between patient experience, patient safety, and clinical effectiveness for a wide range of disease areas, settings, outcome measures, and study designs. It demonstrates positive associations between patient experience and self-rated and objectively measured health outcomes; adherence to recommended clinical practice and medication; preventive care (such as health-promoting behavior, use of screening services and immunization); and resource use (such as hospitalization, length of stay, and primary-care visits). There is some evidence of positive associations between patient experience and measures of the technical quality of care and adverse events."[4]

Now, let's talk about quality from another angle. Consider that evidence-based medicine seeks to reduce variances between clinicians in different parts of the country by benchmarking "best practices" and encouraging their use. To achieve that consistency, it stands to reason that we need great teamwork between physicians and nurses.

A study published by Leslie Curry and colleagues[5] makes that point. The study was designed to look at mortality rates from acute myocardial infarction. The top 5 percent versus the bottom 5 percent in terms of outcomes were investigated in great detail. It was anticipated that evidence-based protocols and standardized guidelines would be responsible for the difference in clinical outcomes. Yet to the investigators' surprise, the differentiating factor was not science at all. Upon careful review, it was found to be more related to the *culture* of the institution. Indeed, "physician champions" and "empowered nurses" had transformed individual units within the hospital and brainstormed their way to better outcomes.

We at Studer Group® find that physician burnout interferes with the interaction of a healthcare team. (This has not been proven in a study, to my knowledge, but I've seen this firsthand.) And having healthcare teams that interact well is a cornerstone of a high-performing culture. We owe it to physicians and staff and—of course—to patients to do all that can be done to reduce burnout.

It can also harm patient perception of care. We've already touched on this issue, above, with the results of the study reported on by Halbesleben and Rathert. Another article—"Is the Professional Satisfaction of General Internists Associated with Patient Satisfaction?" written by Jennifer Haas and colleagues and published in the *Journal of General Internal Medicine*—suggests the converse is also true. The study it features showed that patients under the care of satisfied physicians (satisfied with their profession, to be more precise) reported higher levels of patient satisfaction.[6]

It's worth mentioning here that other studies show satisfied patients are more likely to comply with their medication treatment plan.[7] Obviously, better compliance results in better outcomes—which is just one more piece of evidence that patient perception and clinical quality are intertwined. In my talks, I describe physicians and other providers as behaviorists. The goal is to align the patient's behavior (compliance) to achieve the best possible outcome.

As we discussed earlier in this book, CMS is now using HCAHPS and CG CAHPS results to tie patient perception of care to reimbursement. So this is one more external change that, while not easy, shows how the healthcare payment system is now supporting alignment of providers with value-based purchasing.

It can drive up an organization's recruitment and retention costs. Physicians in general have remarkable "staying power." They can and do weather a lot of adversity while continuing to provide excellent care. However, once burnout reaches a certain level, physicians may simply choose to disengage. They may opt for early retirement, move to part-time employment (already a major trend for physicians), or even leave the practice of medicine altogether. For example, a 2010 survey by the American College of Physicians and the American

Board of Internal Medicine found that one in six general internists had left their field mid-career.[8]

Consider the void created by physicians leaving (or working fewer hours) combined with the growing physician shortage problem and one can see why this is a big problem for organizations. The costs of recruiting a physician can range up to $250,000.[9]

This is not just a problem for individual health systems but for the industry and the nation. As Kieran Walsh, FRCPI, wrote in a letter to the editor in *Academic Medicine*, "The cost of producing a newly graduated doctor in the United States is estimated at $497,000; the cost of producing a fully qualified specialist would be far more. Each time a physician leaves the workforce, this investment is lost."[10]

The reality is that if current physicians remain unhappy, it will be hard to recruit new ones. This is similar to the "nurse burnout" experienced back around 1995 when there was a critical nursing shortage. Yet as a profession, the medical community worked together to fix the problem—and we need to do the same for physicians.

Burnout harms physician productivity and drives up organizational operating costs. We realize intuitively that physicians who are in some phase of burnout, while physically present, may not be working at their full capacity. And there is some evidence that physician productivity is negatively correlated with burnout.[11] Since virtually all healthcare organizations need to become as efficient and effective as possible, this is one more reason to aggressively tackle burnout.

One way to treat burnout and improve productivity is to focus on helping physicians align and engage. (While burnout and lack of engagement may be two separate problems, I have found there is a good amount of overlap in the solutions.) In a *Becker's Hospital Review* article, Tamara Rosin quotes Stephen Moore, MD, CMO, of Houston-based CHI St. Luke's Health, on how today's shifting business model "has really forced healthcare to unify operational and clinical leadership."

"Establishing a highly engaged physician population allows hospitals to more effectively target the quality and efficiency issues that may help to reduce complications, mortality, readmissions, and length of stay," writes Rosin. "It allows the whole hospital business to come together as a team and tackle inefficiencies while addressing the needs of the community and making the patient experience more satisfactory, according to Dr. Moore."[12]

It makes episodes of incivility more likely. The study of incivility is a specialized area in the social sciences that deals with the interactions and perceptions experienced by individuals in the workforce. I see it as a litmus test that shows a workplace is dysfunctional and people are less likely to work together as teams. Christine Pearson and Christine Porath explore this subject in their book, *The Cost of Bad Behavior* (New York, Penguin Books, 2009).

In the book, incivility is defined as "…the exchange of seemingly inconsequential inconsiderate words and deeds that violate conventional norms of workplace conduct." Thus it serves to measure how cohesively workers interact with one another. Examples of incivility would include rudeness, condescension, failure to return calls or respond to questions from coworkers, and generally not interacting in a cooperative fashion.

The magnitude of the problem is epidemic: The authors report that over 95 percent of people have experienced it and over 80 percent believe that it is a problem. They add that 12 percent of workers leave their jobs due to incivility.

CFOs of healthcare organizations will be interested to know that incivility has a significant "cost," quite literally. Pearson and Porath state that rehiring, as a percentage of the employee's salary, can range from 30-50 percent (lower-level), through 150 percent (mid-level), to as high as 400 percent (for high-level employees)! They add that Fortune 1000 executives spend seven weeks of their time on a yearly basis dealing with conflicts between employees.

One of the hospitals for which these consultants worked stated that it cost almost $26,000 just to deal with a single episode of incivility. Another large hospital organization (with yearly revenues of $1 billion) reported that it spent $70 million yearly dealing with incivility. In an age of declining revenues, increasing costs, and the finitude of resources, these funds could be utilized much more wisely.[13]

The 2009 Doctor-Nurse Behavior Survey, reported by the American College of Physician Executives, polled 2,100 clinicians (physicians and nurses). Over 97 percent of the healthcare organizations reported "behavior problems" such as yelling, cursing, degrading comments, and refusing to work together. In 45 percent of the cases the physicians were the culprits, and in 48 percent there was an equal mix of physicians and nurses. Clearly, the pressures that lead to burnout are creating a high-stress work environment that takes its toll on everyone.[14]

It leads to malpractice litigation. We know that compassionate, efficient healthcare results in better patient outcomes and satisfaction. This, in turn, decreases the costs of malpractice litigation. It's just common sense. And physicians who are stressed, depressed, and burned out are far less likely to be able to provide this optimal level of care. (Among other problems, burnout can diminish physician empathy, which blocks the emotional bond required to practice good medicine.)

The connection between on-the-job stress levels and malpractice suits has been demonstrated in a number of studies.[15] Not surprisingly, one study found evidence that physicians with burnout had higher malpractice claims.[16]

It blocks change initiatives from moving through the organization. As our industry's external environment continues to change, health systems will shift and evolve right along with it. The demands placed on them by the government, by private insurers, and by patients themselves will only increase. What this means is that organizations have to become more agile, to improve steadily and continuously, day after day, month after month, year after year. (The escalator is steadily moving downward, so anyone who isn't climbing is descending.)

As health systems strive to hardwire new tactics, fine-tune their processes, and make other needed changes, they want physicians at the table, on board, and fully engaged. *More* than on board, in fact. Physicians are valuable, not just as participants in change but as enthusiastic drivers of change. I believe physicians want the same. If they are not driving change, these efforts at improvement will be short-lived (if they get off the ground at all). When physicians are burned out, they barely have the energy to continue on with "business as usual," much less change the way they interact with patients, staff, and colleagues.

Finally, it dulls the passion and purpose that drives physicians and results in great care. Physicians, like all healthcare professionals, don't view what they do as a job. They see it as a calling. Otherwise, they couldn't do the tough things they have to do every day. Without that passion and sense of purpose driving them, they wouldn't be able to connect with patient after patient in a way that reassures them, inspires them to follow their treatment plan, and ultimately puts them on the path to recovery. They certainly wouldn't be able to see people in pain or deliver the bad news that, inevitably, comes to all of us.

Burnout extinguishes that inner flame that allows physicians to do their important work, to really put their heart and soul into it. Sometimes the conditions that lead to burnout can erode a physician's values (and when you deal with people's lives, compromising your values is a very dangerous thing). We as an industry cannot allow this to happen to physicians.

What's more, we can't allow physician burnout to affect other team members. Health systems are just that—complex, intertwined *systems* of professionals who must communicate and share responsibilities with each other. When one person is impacted by burnout, their exhaustion, cynicism, and sadness touches everyone who comes into contact with them. Their passion and purpose can be affected, too—and, of course, the patient ultimately bears the brunt of the burnout.

So, given all of these issues (and no doubt others not covered in this book), it is obvious even the best-run organization has opportunities to help physicians deal with burnout. As we discussed earlier, until recently physicians have been independent agents. Health systems simply have not had the ability to impact physicians' lives that they have now. Plus, recent industry changes have worsened the burnout problem to the extent that it is as noticeable as it is today.

Finally, a big challenge lies in helping physicians assess their own level of satisfaction. It isn't always easy to tell when someone is burned out. Because of their independent nature, physicians are unlikely to "self-report" or ask for help. In fact, they may see it as unprofessional or as a sign of weakness. This is all the more reason why health systems leaders need to educate themselves on what burnout looks like and what to do when it is recognized in a physician.

In the 1980s, I worked in the behavioral health field. A part of my job was helping supervisors spot early symptoms in employees' behavior and offer them help before the situation became severe. I found that this training helped supervisors better assess what was taking place and led to early discussions, preventing the issue from escalating as well as saving careers.

With 50 percent of physicians, or possibly more, currently dealing with burnout, it is evident that there is much to be gained by helping prevent the escalation of this issue. Disruptive physicians really are a very small group. It makes far more sense to spend our precious time helping and lifting up the majority of physicians than to devote all of our time to a tiny percentage of physicians. (However, like any disruptive employee, disruptive physicians cannot be ignored. What is permitted is promoted.)

What do physicians need? Research shows physicians desire input and inclusion into the decision making that affects their lives and the lives of their patients. They want to work for efficient, effective organizations that consistently provide excellent quality of care. Physicians want clear feedback on what they're doing right and on what needs improving. And yes, reward and recognition is nice—not because they crave praise and glory but because it is always nice to know when one is making a difference.

Knowing what physicians want and providing it will go a long way toward alleviating physician burnout. And we can go even further.

More and more regulations are affecting health systems. More and more demands are being placed on them. More and more reimbursement is being tied to outcomes. We're living and working in tough times, and there is just no way that a workforce of clinicians diminished in number and functionality can deal with the burden of higher volume and acuity of patient needs.

Something has to give. In my mind, those systems that are best able to deal with the epidemic of burnout will be the same ones that are able to engage their physicians in powerful and new ways.

Physicians, even when manifesting signs of burnout, have a deep reservoir of passion for their profession. Healthcare leaders recognize the need to invest the resources that are required to retain these valuable caregivers. There are simply not enough resources or time to recruit a new generation of clinicians. Saving this generation is job number one.

Just as we have a sacred trust to provide the best possible care for patients, we have one to help physicians restore their passion and reignite their sense of purpose. Right now too many are on autopilot. We need to help them relight the "pilot light," and we can do this by identifying burnout, naming it, treating it, and reconnecting these physicians to passion and purpose.

PART THREE:

RECOGNIZING PHYSICIAN BURNOUT

CHAPTER SEVEN:

A FEW "RED FLAGS" TO WATCH FOR: BURNOUT SIGNS AND SYMPTOMS FOR LEADERS AND PHYSICIANS

What is burnout, anyway? Before we can talk about symptoms, and then later about treatment, let's define the condition. A simple definition could be expressed as the "progressive loss of idealism, energy, and purpose."[1]

Psychologist Christina Maslach codified burnout in the MBI (Maslach Burnout Inventory). This 22-item inventory is broken down into three dimensions: Emotional Exhaustion, Cynicism, and Ineffectiveness. It has been the validated tool and gold standard for measuring burnout since the 1970s.

Here's a brief description of these three dimensions the survey covers:

- **Emotional Exhaustion.** This is the sense of being emotionally drained while working with other people and the dread that accompanies thoughts of having to go to work. Rather than being energized by one's job, one is exhausted by it. It's the loss of the "passion" that's so fundamental to providing excellent healthcare.

- **Cynicism.** I've also seen this expressed as depersonalization, withdrawal, and compassion fatigue. In short, the burned out person becomes numb to the humanity of others. In medicine this manifests as the physician no longer regarding the patient as a unique individual with fears, needs, and hopes. The patient becomes another "number," or just another member of a disease group (diabetic, hypertensive, etc.). The heart becomes "hardened," and empathy is lost.

- **Ineffectiveness/Lack of Efficacy.** What we're talking about here is the loss of one's desire to accomplish great goals and make the world a better place. This is very serious, as physicians (much like nurses, teachers, ministers, and counselors) by their nature want to serve. The burned out clinician, who started out with such idealism, really begins to doubt that their work has purpose and that they are able to make a difference.

Below is a sample question from each of the dimensions found in the MBI:

- **Emotional Exhaustion:**
  1. I feel burned out from my work.

- **Cynicism:**
  10. I have become more callous toward people since I took this job.

- **Ineffectiveness/Lack of Efficacy:**
  21. In my work, I deal with emotional problems very calmly.

To access the full inventory of questions, please visit http://www.mindgarden.com/117-maslach-burnout-inventory.[2]

In his book *Transforming Burnout: A Simple Guide to Self-Renewal*, Alan Shelton, MD, describes his own journey with burnout. In one passage he writes:

"At a recent conference I heard one physician say, 'One cool autumn afternoon with all the exam rooms occupied, and with my waiting room full, I quietly slipped out the back door.' I knew just what he meant. Even though I had never given into this impulse when I was suffering from burnout, I vividly remember that powerful desire to escape from work."[3]

No one in any field *wants* to experience burnout. No one wants to escape what they do for a living. It's a terrible and debilitating feeling. But it may be worse for physicians than for people in many other professions. If you're a physician, you didn't just happen into medicine by chance or settle on it as a second- or third-choice career. What's more, you're probably a perfectionist, an idealist, a tireless worker, and a believer in "callings." (All these traits make physicians uniquely susceptible for burnout, and they may also make it more painful.)

Imagine you've invested many years and hundreds of thousands of dollars to become a doctor and you have a burning desire to help people. So discovering that you are unhappy, losing your empathy for patients, and believing (however wrongly) that you really *can't* help them is a crushing blow. It's devastating. Remember, it's not easy psychologically or financially to change careers when you're established as a physician and especially when you're burdened with lots of debt.

It's no wonder that, as we've discussed earlier, physician burnout is so prevalent. I've seen statistics ranging from 25 percent all the way up to 60 percent.[4] It's impossible to get a precise statistic since burnout isn't always a clear-cut issue and also since so few physicians are likely to self-report. I'd say it's probably safe to estimate that one of every two physicians is, has been, or will be burned out.

So it's important to know: What does physician burnout look like? What are its signs and symptoms? To make the task of writing this a bit easier, I'm going to assume you're a health system leader or a clinician wanting to recognize burnout in the physicians you work with. (Of course I know this won't be true for every reader.

If you're a physician, I urge you to read these with an eye toward recognizing the signs of burnout in yourself and colleagues.)

The Burnout Spectrum: How It Manifests

No one is fine one day and burned out the next. It happens gradually over time. It's like coming down with a bad cold. First there is a little sniffle, maybe a little scratch in the throat, a feeling of being tired. A couple days later, the throat is burning, the nose is running, the head is aching, and you're feverish. Sometimes you end up with a bacterial infection that you have to treat with antibiotics.

In much the same way, burnout may begin with subtle symptoms. Maybe a physician is too tired to see extra patients. Maybe they're not as open to a patient's point of view. Maybe they don't take the time to make that extra phone call (the one they would have previously made right away). These are leading indicators of burnout.

Later, though, the physician may begin to exhibit irritability or even outright anger. Maybe their relationships begin to suffer. Maybe they even fall into a deep depression, develop a substance abuse problem, or start to get sued for malpractice. These are lagging indicators of burnout.

Remember, burnout is the opposite of engagement, so a burned out physician will surely not be working at full capacity, even if they think they are. While most physicians will try their best to care for their patients, they will most likely *not* have the energy or enthusiasm needed to implement new tactics that health system leaders want them to implement.

Most experts agree that you can't shorten the duration of a cold (it just has to run its course), but I believe that, in general, one can halt the progression of burnout.

It doesn't *have* to progress to the dangerous, even deadly phases where broken relationships, substance abuse, and even suicide can occur.

The good news is that there are plenty of things organizations can do to help physicians avoid and recover from burnout (and we'll discuss them in Part 4 of this book). But in the meantime, here are some red flags that need to be watched for—and the sooner flags are spotted the better. It is better to catch when yellow versus red.

Leading Indicators of Physician Burnout

The physician exhibits the Three Ds: Disengagement, Disinterest, and Disconnection. When a physician seems reluctant to attend meetings, participate in change initiatives, embrace tactics that others around them are embracing, or even discuss critical issues, it may be an early sign of burnout.

There's a noticeable loss of passion. Of course, personalities are different. Some people may be more enthusiastic, cheerful, and energetic than others by nature.

But even in people who are more low-key, burnout can manifest as a blunting of one's personality and emotional energy. They may seem quieter, apathetic, tired, and even visibly sad or anxious. It's like their "get up and go" has gotten up and gone.

Work habits change. A physician in the early stages of burnout may start missing meetings when previously they have always attended them. They may work fewer hours, come in late, or leave early. Or perhaps they stop taking time to communicate with nurses and other staff members on things they need to know.

There is less energy. They may seem obviously tired or complain of being tired. Perhaps they say they are having trouble sleeping. In fact, they may cite tiredness as a reason for seeing fewer patients.

The patient experience starts to suffer. Often, patients are the first ones to notice that a physician is burned out, though they may not realize that's what's wrong. Patients may notice that the physician seems detached, less compassionate than usual, and less responsive to their input.

The physician may start making cynical comments. For instance, you might overhear physicians making unkind or denigrating comments about individual patients or certain patient populations. Or they might aim their cynical remarks at nurses or health system leadership.

They seem irritable or angry, or may lash out. Physicians may sometimes snap at nurses and other staff members. Even if their behavior can't truly be described as "disruptive" (i.e., they're not being verbally abusive or throwing charts around), they may be perpetually short-tempered, sarcastic, or negative.

The physician may often appear to be anxious or fearful. Perhaps they seem nervous, jittery, ill at ease, or have trouble concentrating. Anxiety may also manifest as physical health problems like headaches, insomnia, stomach issues, etc.

They are increasingly dissatisfied with their work and their life in general. While they may not openly announce this (except perhaps in physician satisfaction surveys), it's often apparent in little things they say and do—or don't say and do.

Lagging Indicators of Physician Burnout

The physician may exhibit or express a sense of powerlessness. They may openly say things like, "I feel like a cog in a machine," or, "I have no control over anything anymore…there's no point in even trying." Even if they don't openly state such things, their feelings may be obvious by their total lack of engagement.

They feel a diminished sense of personal accomplishment. This is the lack of efficacy I mentioned earlier. Outside observers may not always be able to tell physicians have stopped being proud of their work, but sometimes they may say things like, "Nothing I do matters," or, "I don't even know why I come to work anymore." (I've actually read that this tends to happen more in female physicians than male ones.)

The physician may withdraw or isolate him/ herself. A burned out physician may avoid colleagues at work and "hide out" in their office. In their personal life, they may begin to avoid friends and even family members and may neglect outside interests for which they had previously shown a lot of enthusiasm. Since physicians tend to define themselves by their work, when they're not feeling good about it, they want to minimize community visibility.

They may become the target of malpractice suits. As we've discussed already, there is a connection between malpractice claims and physician burnout. This makes sense, as physicians with signs of burnout make more medical mistakes.

The physician's personal relationships may crumble. The same conditions that lead to burnout are also hard on personal relationships—especially if the physician tends to internalize things. When you're overworked, stressed out, and bombarded with challenges that seem to have no solution, it's tough to come home and be an attentive, engaged, and loving partner. The physical and emotional issues that come with burnout (exhaustion, insomnia, anxiety, anger) don't help either. Even if they don't end up divorced, the burned out physician may end up feeling lonely and misunderstood inside their marriage.

All the same problems may also ripple through the physician's relationships with kids, extended family, and friends, as well.

They may succumb to substance abuse or serious depression. If burnout goes untreated, a physician may be more prone to using alcohol or other substances (like illicit drugs or even food) to cope with the emotional pain. Also, burnout left untreated often leads to clinical depression. And because substance abuse and clinical depression often feed into each other, physicians can end up struggling with this "double whammy," which is a serious and sometimes even fatal combination.

The Most Frightening Risk of All: Physician Suicide

It's well known that suicide rates among physicians are higher than the general population. In fact, it's believed that physicians are more than twice as likely to kill themselves as compared to people in other professions, and that female physicians are even more likely to do so than males.[5] Specifically, it has been widely reported that between 300 and 400 physicians kill themselves every year.

These are shocking numbers. When you consider the fact that physicians (especially male physicians) are less likely to ask for help, it's clear that organizations need to keep a sharp eye on physicians who seem depressed or severely burned out.

Here, reproduced directly from the American Foundation for Suicide Prevention, are some red flags to watch out for:

Suicide Warning Signs

People who kill themselves exhibit one or more warning signs, either through what they say or what they do. The more warning signs, the greater the risk.

Talk

If a person talks about:

Killing themselves.

Having no reason to live.

Being a burden to others.

Feeling trapped.

Unbearable pain.

Behavior

A person's suicide risk is greater if a behavior is new or has increased, especially if it's related to a painful event, loss, or change.

Increased use of alcohol or drugs.

Looking for a way to kill themselves, such as searching online for materials or means.

Acting recklessly.

Withdrawing from activities.

Isolating from family and friends.

Sleeping too much or too little.

Visiting or calling people to say goodbye.

Giving away prized possessions.

Aggression.

Mood

People who are considering suicide often display one or more of the following moods.

Depression.

Loss of interest.

Rage.

Irritability.

Humiliation.

Anxiety.[6]

There are no easy answers for preventing physician suicide. However, I recommend that leaders do the following:

1. Talk openly about the problem of physician suicide inside your organization. Help leaders and all team members recognize the warning signs. By talking about it, we not only educate but also destigmatize the subject so that people will be

more likely to report suicidal feelings in themselves and others.

2. Emphasize to physicians that it is absolutely crucial that they report feelings of hopelessness or any suicidal thoughts to a leader or a mental health professional. Assure them that they will not be penalized in any way and that you'll assist them in getting the help they need.

3. Reach out to any physician (or anyone else) you suspect is troubled or suffering from severe burnout. Tell all leaders and staff members to do the same. Don't worry about offending or embarrassing the individual—it is better to take the risk and save a life than to remain silent and be sorry later.

4. Finally, do everything you possibly can to create the kind of environment where physicians can feel engaged and thrive professionally and emotionally. It's far better to proactively shore up the mental, emotional, and spiritual health of physicians than to try to help them once they are already suicidal. (This, of course, is the aim of this book.)

If you are a physician reading this and are feeling suicidal, I say: Please seek help right away. Call the National Suicide Prevention Lifeline at 1-800-273-8255 or speak to a trusted colleague or mental health professional. I promise...things *can and will* get better and you *can and will* be able to recapture (or perhaps experience for the first time) the joy and fulfillment that come from being a fully engaged physician. At the very least, you *can and will* be able to move to a different position or work environment where you can use your gifts in a way that helps others and that is more conducive to your own well-being and happiness.

The signs and symptoms of burnout are not always easy to spot. However, taking steps to familiarize ourselves, our leadership teams, and our entire staff with the indicators covered in this chapter can go a long way toward creating an organization-wide culture where people are constantly on the lookout for this problem.

In fact, beyond building this broad and deep awareness, we probably don't need to invest more resources in identifying those who are burned out. After all, we already know that burnout may affect one out of every two physicians. What we do need to do is create the kind of environment where physicians and everyone else know that it's safe for them to discuss this topic and seek help for it.

The rest of this book will be dedicated to actions organizations can start implementing right away to get physicians engaged and aligned. Remember, an engaged physician is less likely to be a burned out physician since the two states of being are opposites. When we do all that is in our power to create the best possible environment for physicians to practice medicine, everyone wins—the physicians themselves, yes, but also the entire healthcare team, the patients, and the health system itself.

PART FOUR:

We Are All in This Together: Tools and Tactics for Treating Physician Burnout

Before one can begin to tackle the problem of physician burnout, it is vital to know what drives physicians in the first place. If physicians are burning out in large part because they are *not* getting their basic wants and needs met—and this is probably a safe assumption—then any help we as healthcare system leaders can provide has to flow from a solid understanding of what makes these men and women tick. In my book *Results That Last*, I talk about this in terms of learning the person's "what."

To be clear, here we are referring to "needs and wants" that healthcare system leaders have influence over. We *cannot* control whether physicians exercise, get enough rest, eat a healthful diet, get in touch with their spirituality, nurture personal relationships, etc. We can encourage them to do these things and even make resources available to assist with them, but these are largely self-help measures. (We'll address these later on.) But for now, when we talk about physician drivers, we're talking about things physicians want and need in the workplace.

That said, there are four big, overarching physician drivers. These are:

FIGURE IV.1	PHYSICIAN DRIVERS	
Physician Driver	**Action**
Quality	Physicians want to know their patients are receiving excellent clinical care and a great patient experience.
Efficiency	Physicians want to work with people who have the information needed at hand to discuss their patients. When we can help a physician maximize efficiency, over the course of a day we will be able to save them 30 minutes or more.
Input	Physicians need a seat at the table so they can provide input when decisions are being made that affect clinical outcomes and operations.
Appreciation	Physicians value a "thank you" and acknowledgment. Too often people forget to show gratitude to physicians, so when we take the time to do so, it really means a lot. They also want to see follow-up on their input in the form of tangible change (this is also a form of appreciation and respect).

Now, let's talk a bit more about each of these drivers, one at a time.

PHYSICIAN DRIVER #1: QUALITY. Of the four physician drivers, the one physicians care most about is the quality of care that's provided to their patients. This is true whether we're talking about an inpatient setting, an outpatient setting, or a population health scenario in which a physician is managing the health of thousands of people.

To physicians, "quality care" doesn't refer only to the brief period of time the patient is in their office. It also refers to the length of time from the patient call to make their appointment to when they walk into the office…to what happens when they finally see the receptionist…to how smoothly any tests go…to how long it takes to get test results back…to how the patient experiences the billing process.

Of course, it also refers to how quickly the treatment plan starts to work and the patient gets better and, if they have to be hospitalized, how well their stay goes and how the subsequent recovery progresses. This even includes when inpatient care is managed by hospitalists.

In other words, physicians care about the quality of much more than just the time they spend face-to-face with the patient. They care about everything *around* that window of time—everything before, everything during, and everything after it. It all impacts the patient's perception of the physician and, more important, the patient's outcome.

Well-trained staff and low turnover are also integral to quality (as well as the next physician driver, efficiency). Doctors want a team they can count on. That's why they need to be kept informed about hiring and onboarding plans. In fact, they should be invited to be part of the interview process.

PHYSICIAN DRIVER #2: EFFICIENCY. Physicians care about having an efficient, effective work environment. They know that they've got to keep moving at all times. They know that patients are waiting to see them. Unlike other professions where people can say, "I can't see you today," or, "I have to change my schedule," physicians understand that patients have a serious, urgent need to see them.

I was recently talking to a non-healthcare professional. I said, "If you were working and somebody told you that your child fell on the playground and had a bump on his head, what would you do?" The person said, "I'd immediately go to the school." Most people would. But if you're a physician with eight people in the reception area waiting to see you, some of them very concerned about their health, how easy is it to leave? You're constantly caught in between balancing your personal life and your professional life.

Of course, if the organization you're working for—whether it's a private practice or a huge academic medical center—is efficient and effective, it doesn't solve the issue of your child falling and needing you. However, it does help you feel better about the fact that you don't have wasted time. Physicians, like everyone else, want to use their time wisely. An effective and efficient operation is about more than creating great patient flow. That's part of it but not all. We want to make it cost effective but we also want to make it respectful of the physician's time.

When organizations can't satisfy this driver, the physician may think that operations are not efficient and not effective, but they may also think, *They don't respect my time*. It's particularly difficult when a physician is being evaluated on a production model evaluation tool. The physician will say (or at least think), "I'm working as hard as I can, but things around me that I can't control are working against me." This very much leaves a physician feeling like a hamster on a wheel in a cage.

Physicians often feel they can't quit their job. Many healthcare professionals, if they're unhappy, can leave the field. They might not make as much money or have such great benefits in a different job, but often they can leave without a huge drop in their lifestyle. But the physician probably has a large debt load, is involved in the community, has a medical license for that state, and is already approved by the insurance providers.

So when physicians are unhappy, they stay, which makes it difficult for them and for everyone else. The key is creating an environment where a physician can be a much happier person—and so can everyone around them.

All departments play a role here—Environmental Services for cleanliness, Nutritional Services for providing food, Information Technology for help with EMRs, etc. Everyone contributes to fewer workarounds, efficient medical supply and ordering processes, surgical blocks that work, and scheduling software that works between office and hospital/procedure. Everyone has a part in creating the right environment.

PHYSICIAN DRIVER #3: INPUT. I was meeting with an organization, and a leader asked me, "How do you align physicians?" I said, "Physicians are smart people. You ask them how they would like to be aligned."

I believe the best approach is also the simplest: Bring physicians into the room and say, "This is where the organization needs to be by such and such a date. How can we get there?"

After a few meetings, the physicians are going to lock in because they want the organization they work with to be successful. Sure, there may be some conversations that get off-kilter as everyone gets to know each other. Maybe we have to solve some other issues. But in the long run, physicians want input because they have skin in the game, particularly as the environment leads to a more integrated healthcare system. They *want* the organization to do well.

My father worked at General Motors for 41 years. He was not in the car/automobile division—he worked in another part of the organization—yet we also had General Motors cars. Whenever he saw a relative without one, he would urge them to buy a GM car. Why? Because he saw that if somebody bought a GM car, it positively impacted his job security.

Physicians understand that the better the organization does, the better they personally do. That means we have to meet with physicians to tell them where the organization is going, what the overall goals are, and what the physician's goals are—but we also need to ask the physician how we can get there.

Here's a recent situation that relates to the power of input. The CEO of a rather large healthcare system told me they were doing a physician retreat and asked for my thoughts. I already knew a little bit about this organization; their physician engagement results were poor. So I said, "Why don't you try this? Why don't you just break them into small groups around the table, give each group a flip chart, and facilitate? Ask: 'What do you like about practicing medicine here? What is it that we do well so that we can keep doing it and reinforce doing it?'" So the groups broke up and did a very nice job. Actually, they ended up with a longer list than the administration expected. Results were then shared and this created a nice, positive tone.

Then they moved into: "What are the opportunities for improvement?" The conversation shifted to what the healthcare system can and can't control. The physicians got very engaged again, and they came up with a big list of things they thought could be going better. One of them was a better referral system. Another one had to do with the "printing approval committee" and how it was preventing a physician from getting a needed printer. So some were easier fixes than others, but basically they listed opportunities for improvement.

What they did during this meeting of physicians was introduce a practice called nominal voting. Some people knew it; others didn't. Basically, every physician had so many votes that they could cast. When they were done voting, they prioritized the issues that were most important to them.

What this did was truly give physicians as a group a feeling of inclusion, a feeling of input, a feeling of skin in the game, a feeling of "We're all in this together." Once a physician has more input into a new tactic or process, they're also going to have more of a commitment to make it successful. This has always been the case, but in a time when physicians are feeling such a tremendous loss of control, input is more powerful than ever. It builds that initial foundation of trust that is the cornerstone of success.

PHYSICIAN DRIVER #4: APPRECIATION. Physicians appreciate reinforcement, encouragement, and reward and recognition. It's easy to fall into the trap of thinking that a physician might not need reward and recognition. Why? Because people already admire them and treat them with respect. Also, they did well in school and they do well in life. Finally, we may think they probably get lots of appreciation from patients already.

I'm sure all of this is true. But what we have to remember is that physicians also get big "withdrawals" in this area, particularly with patients they can't cure or patients who have to hear a tough message that the physician might not want to give. Physicians need more appreciation and more reward and recognition just to balance out these really difficult moments in their lives. This is why it's so important to look for methods to provide reward and recognition.

Years ago when I was working at an organization, a horrific accident happened, and a number of patients were brought to the Emergency Department and rushed into surgery. There were so many healthcare professionals needed in the surgery rooms that it was impossible for nurses to come out and update the families on what was going on. One of the radiologists happened to be in that area and saw the challenge they had, and, on his own, decided to be the liaison between what was happening in surgery and the family members in the waiting room.

We'd heard about this from the staff and also from some of the families. It was unusual because it was apparent that this radiologist wasn't normally in that area. He just happened to be walking by, saw a problem, and brought the solution. Anyway, his peers felt he deserved special recognition for going "above and beyond" this way.

Every month that the department had meetings, we would recognize certain employees and certain leaders by naming them "Employee of the Month." The Radiology Department nominated this person, and even though he was contracted through a radiology group, we named him our Employee of the Month. So when he came to the meeting, we told this story, and then we gave him a gift. A number of radiological technologists ran out with confetti and horns and poppers and made a big deal about it and then went back to work. It was a wonderful experience.

What got me was the next week I received a letter from that physician. He told me in all the years of practicing medicine, that celebration was one of the best moments of his life. Don't underestimate the difference reward and recognition makes for people.

I have been fortunate to work with wonderful physicians. One was a neurosurgeon named Troy Tippett. In my book *Hardwiring Excellence*, I tell the story of the Wow Program and how one of the unit coordinators had given him a Wow card. This really had little monetary value. If you got five of them, you could go to the gift shop and you could get something. Anyway, the unit coordinator was pretty excited. In fact, she got a real thrill out of giving Dr. Tippett a Wow card. I thought that was nice and I felt good for the unit coordinator. But I underestimated the impact that would have on him.

A couple of months later, I happened to be in Dr. Tippett's office. When I looked up, I saw his medical degrees, I saw pictures of his family, and there, stuck to his wall in between his medical degrees, was that Wow award. I realized it had meant a lot to Dr. Tippett because it came from someone he worked with. Again, never underestimate what appreciation does for physicians.

A Quick Overview of the Tactics in Part 4

If we know that physicians care about these four things—quality of care, efficiency and effectiveness, input, and appreciation—it stands to reason to implement techniques around them. This engages physicians and at the same time works to alleviate and prevent burnout. We will also look at the techniques that provide development for physicians. After all, we don't just want their input but also their solutions, and we want their contribution to be as impactful as possible.

Part 4 will outline the Diagnostic, Measurement, and Treatment Strategies, which are Tools and Tactics for getting physicians engaged to reduce and eliminate burnout. Also provided are what I am calling "out of the box" strategies and tactics. These are unusual or unconventional ideas that organizations don't typically consider—or perhaps ideas they have considered or even implemented but not on a level that maximizes their impact. (See Figure IV.2)

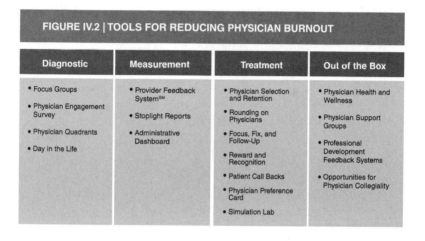

FIGURE IV.2 | TOOLS FOR REDUCING PHYSICIAN BURNOUT

Diagnostic	Measurement	Treatment	Out of the Box
• Focus Groups • Physician Engagement Survey • Physician Quadrants • Day in the Life	• Provider Feedback System℠ • Stoplight Reports • Administrative Dashboard	• Physician Selection and Retention • Rounding on Physicians • Focus, Fix, and Follow-Up • Reward and Recognition • Patient Call Backs • Physician Preference Card • Simulation Lab	• Physician Health and Wellness • Physician Support Groups • Professional Development Feedback Systems • Opportunities for Physician Collegiality

Finally, there is a chapter called "Physician, Heal Thyself," which provides tactics physicians themselves can use to alleviate burnout and improve their own lives in general.

My hope is that healthcare systems will implement as many of these tactics as possible (and, of course, encourage physicians to find ways to heal their own burnout). I know you may not be able to hardwire all of these tactics right away, but may start with one or two from each category. I am hopeful that once you start seeing results, you'll want to implement the others. Also, I urge you to customize your plan to fit your physicians' individual needs.

As you can see from the slide below, taken from the Medscape Physician Lifestyle Report 2015, physicians experience burnout at different rates depending on their age range.

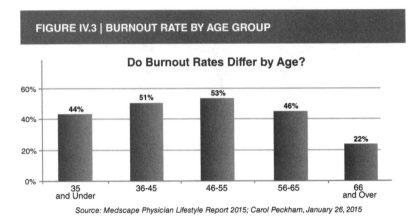

FIGURE IV.3 | BURNOUT RATE BY AGE GROUP

Do Burnout Rates Differ by Age?

Source: Medscape Physician Lifestyle Report 2015; Carol Peckham, January 26, 2015

Burnout rates are lowest in the youngest and oldest physicians. Yet, in the youngest category, they are still surprisingly high. Of all the physicians under 35 surveyed for the Medscape Physician Lifestyle Report, 44 percent reported that they were burned out.

It appears that burnout peaks in mid-life. Over half of physicians in this age range reported being burned out (51 percent of those between 36 and 45 years of age, and 53 percent between ages 46 and 55), while rates declined to 22 percent in physicians 66 and over.

The drivers of burnout differ by age range. For example, younger physicians who still have a lot of medical school debt might be feeling major financial pressures. They may also be dealing with time management issues. Middle-aged physicians may be struggling with "sandwich generation" issues like raising kids while also helping care for aging parents—and, perhaps, having a tougher time dealing with all the changes happening around them than their younger colleagues. Older physicians might be struggling with technology changes, as well as searching for a sense of purpose and fulfillment.

Keep these differences in mind as you create your organization's burnout treatment plan. For example, you might offer younger physicians financial counseling and provide time management classes and support groups for your middle-aged ones. You might also provide extra training to physicians who seem to be having a lot of trouble switching to electronic medical records or coping with some other aspect of the changing healthcare environment.

In other words, as much as you can, tailor your "burnout prescription" to the individual needs of the physician.

CHAPTER EIGHT:

ORGANIZATIONAL DIAGNOSTIC TOOLS

P hysicians are key stakeholders in any healthcare organization. In working with an organization, I asked the senior leadership team, "What is your revenue?" They replied that it was in the neighborhood of $700 million. I asked, "How much is based on the work of physicians?" They said, "All of it."

Almost 100 percent of an organization's revenue originates with physicians. Healthcare leaders, like all leaders in any industry, want to learn everything they can learn about these key stakeholders. The good news is that there are techniques that can be used to learn more about what physicians are thinking and feeling.

Just as there's no expensive, fancy piece of technology to get physicians engaged, there's no perfect high-tech way to find out if they are disengaged. It would be much easier if there were a switch to flip or a button to press. Sure, technology can validate what is done, but conversation and follow-up are the key ingredients: the give and take of sharing information and listening carefully to each other.

This is no different from the skills physicians use when they diagnose a patient. Listening is a big part of a clinical diagnosis, and it also plays a big role in leaders' efforts to diagnose what's going on with physicians. In other words, as one seeks to engage physicians and alleviate and prevent burnout, one needs to hone and perfect their "human skills."

Let's go over some techniques that can help diagnose how physicians are feeling while seeking to create a better practice environment.

Focus Groups

Focus groups have been used in healthcare for years. They add value as the group setting triggers ideas that might not otherwise come to the surface. Person A might say something that sparks a thought in Person B; then Person C might chime in with the same concern or maybe a different take on it. People bounce ideas off each other and build on other participants' solutions. There's valuable synergy.

When I was president of a hospital, focus groups with physicians proved very helpful. These are more formal than saying, "Come down and have breakfast with two or three administrators." Literally, we sat down with small groups of physicians, much like I talked about earlier.

Questions were asked like *What do we do well? What could we do better? What could really improve patient care? What can make your work environment better?* These are techniques that worked.

At the time, one of the big concerns was nursing. And as the issue was broken down, it was realized that nursing retention was at the heart of it. Selection and retention of talent was not done well, and our reliance was based on what the physicians felt was too much agency nursing. While agency nurses can be very valuable, research shows that low employee turnover improves process improvement, length of stay, and mortality data, which means better clinical outcomes. And so it was shared with the physicians that the number-one goal was to reduce agency nursing. Also covered was what they could do to help retain nurses.

There is a real art to focus groups. It's more complicated than it sounds. But I will offer a few tips for holding successful physician focus groups:

1. Figure out a convenient time and place. Make it as easy as possible for the physicians you're inviting. You don't want to interfere with their (already challenging) work time, but you also don't want them to have to come in on their day off.

2. Carefully select your participants. There should be six to eight physicians per focus group. Fewer than four is too few; more than twelve is too many. You'll want to give them a couple weeks' notice to make it convenient for them.

3. Choose a great facilitator. You'll want someone who is "neutral" so people won't be afraid to speak up. They should be knowledgeable on the topic at hand and skilled at engaging people. I have seen some healthcare leaders also facilitate these groups well.

4. Ask the right questions. In addition to ones I shared earlier, ask questions specific to your organization.

5. Afterward, communicate the results—and if possible, take action on a solution. If physicians are already feeling cynical, you don't want this to seem like a pointless exercise. You really want to get a quick "win" if you're to get them engaged.

Physician Engagement Survey

This survey, sometimes called a physician satisfaction survey, is one of the best diagnostic tools for providing insight into issues like quality, efficiency, and input. More specifically, outcomes reveal how physicians feel about some of the services in a healthcare system—the Emergency, Pathology, Radiology, Surgery, and other departments, the hospitalists, and so on.

It asks the physician, by specialty, how they feel about certain departments and services that are provided to them: Registration, Billing, Imaging, Laboratory, Nursing, and so on. It includes some general questions about the direction of the organization and how much trust physicians have in the senior administration to be responsive. Outcomes will also point to those behaviors and actions that build trust. What builds trust, of course, is fixing things, following through, responsiveness—which is why it's so vital to take action on what is revealed by the survey.

Think of the physician engagement survey as a key diagnostic tool for engagement—like an MRI or CT scan. The data tells where the focus needs to be, where there are no problems or issues, and where there are. Where there is a problem or an issue, the engagement survey helps prioritize which actions to take first.

An additional point is to determine the frequency with which the survey should be deployed. This will depend on the level of importance that you place on physician satisfaction. At minimum, a formal survey should be deployed annually, with small, focused, and/or informal surveying occurring more frequently. If the organization has low physician satisfaction, a decision may be made to formally conduct a survey more often. (Studer Group® has found that organizations with satisfaction issues often do not measure it frequently enough.)

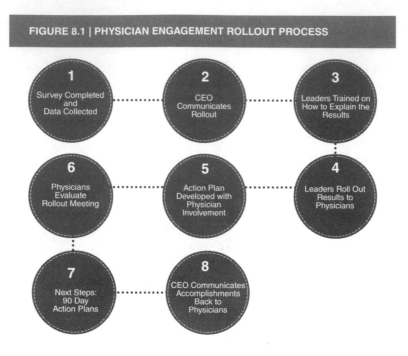

FIGURE 8.1 | PHYSICIAN ENGAGEMENT ROLLOUT PROCESS

Physician Quadrants

When my book *Results That Last* hit the *Wall Street Journal* bestseller list, I was asked to speak at non-healthcare companies. In conversations with their leaders, it quickly became apparent the most successful companies had deep insight regarding which customers represented their various revenue streams, their likes and dislikes, the status of the current relationship, etc. And while physicians may or may not fit the description of "customer," they do represent the largest impact on revenue—so health systems will want to have a similar depth of knowledge about them

To help organizations have a more structured way to assess alignment, the Physician Quadrant tool was created.

The first step in using this tool is to identify the physicians who have the most influence on operations (based on their role, their impact on revenue, etc.). Then divide this group into four quadrants based upon their level of alignment with the organization. (Keep in mind that alignment is different from performance, although performance does factor in.)

Next, label the quadrants as (1) "Loyal"; (2) "Want to Be Aligned"; (3) "Skeptical"; and (4) "Naysayer." Alternately, you might follow the lead of one organization that chose to change the labels to (1) "Always"; (2) "Often"; (3) "Sometimes"; and (4) "Never."

Finally, place every name on your "influential physicians" list into one of the four quadrants. Let's look at each quadrant and what it represents. (See Figure 8.2.)

Quadrant 1: "Loyal" (Always)

These are the "go to" physicians. When we want to have somebody talk to a potential physician coming into our system, these are the people we want to meet with them. These are the physicians who are inherently supportive. They see the value in the changes the organization is making and will actively support those changes.

Key Actions to Take with Quadrant 1 Physicians Include:

- Thank physicians for their support at a group or individual meeting.
- Ask what the system does well.
- Ask about and focus on key operational issues that if fixed would make their work better.
- Send a note to all the departments complimented by the physicians, giving credit to the physicians for sharing this recognition.

Quadrant 2: "Want to Be Aligned" (Often)

Physicians placed in Quadrant 2 are those who want to be on board and are most of the time, but there are one or two things that might be bothering them that keep them from being fully aligned with system leaders. Maybe it's an operational or political issue or frustration with a particular individual. Whatever the issue, something isn't working as well as they would like. It's like they have a pebble in their shoe. They're going to walk with you, but not nearly as quickly as the physicians without the pebble. Our goal with them is to help them get that pebble out of the shoe.

If operations are improved, Quadrant 2 physicians will move to Quadrant 1 in probably anywhere from six months to a year. When this critical mass of physicians is moved, it will help the rest of the organization move forward as well.

Key Actions to Take with Quadrant 2 Physicians Include:

- Use the same actions as with Quadrant 1 physicians.
- If you cannot address a concern, say so and explain why. Physicians would rather hear a "no" than be left in limbo.

Note that Quadrants 1 and 2 will most likely represent 60 percent or more of the physicians practicing medicine in a given system.

Quadrant 3: "Skeptical" (Sometimes)

These physicians are skeptical. They have many issues and concerns. While they are sometimes supportive, it is highly variable. The organization will need to be relentless to move them; it takes time, but they can be moved.

Normally what moves Quadrant 3 physicians is better operational performance. Many of these physicians have concerns that have built up through the years. It's not just one or two issues. It's not an irritating pebble in the shoe they're dealing with, but rather a jagged rock that's causing a lot of discomfort. They're going to walk very slowly. At times, they're not going to walk at all.

When a physician is in Quadrant 3, it will take anywhere from one year to three years to move them to Quadrant 1 or 2. Even if all fixes are completed, they don't trust it's going to stay fixed. And of course, it's the "stay fixed" that physicians are looking for. This is why it's so important to inquire about operational issues that if improved would make their work environment better. It is also a good time to have frank discussions regarding operational issues that cannot be fixed at all or in the timeframe they would like.

For example, I was working with an organization whose physician offices were originally built and located right next to the hospital campus. Over the years, the neighborhood had changed dramatically, and the geographic area closest to the hospital and medical group had a payer mix that was not the most optimal for a healthcare system. The physicians voiced unhappiness about the payer mix due to the location of their medical offices as they felt more affluent patients didn't live nearby and were reluctant to drive into that area. While years ago the payer mix was not an issue, it was now.

In looking at solutions, mid-term and long-term options were suggested to deal with the issue. A mid-term solution included figuring out how to improve the organization's quality and reputation so much that more affluent patients would be willing to drive to the medical offices and hospital, even though it wasn't close to their homes. A long-term solution included expansion of their outreach, opening up other satellite offices outside the immediate geographic area to the more affluent area.

So while this is an extreme example, it is meant to show that even big challenges can be addressed. The lesson here is "Don't give up." It may take some time, but you will eventually move these physicians' level of trust.

Key Actions to Take with Quadrant 3 Physicians Include:

- Use the same actions as with Quadrants 1 and 2 physicians.

- Have frank discussions regarding operational issues that cannot be fixed at all or in the timeframe they would like.

- Be especially persistent in capturing wins, as this group will have more concerns.

Quadrant 4: "Naysayer" (Never)

These physicians will most likely never be on board. Some are less difficult than others, of course. While you take action to provide these physicians with an excellent work environment, know they likely will never move to Quadrants 1 or 2.

With this in mind, create the right work environment for the benefit of all physicians. A healthcare provider will always want to fix what can be fixed. So, ask the Quadrant 4 physician what is going well and for improvement suggestions regarding operational issues. Stay away from the temptation of thinking when things are fixed, the Quadrant 4 doctor will automatically align and move to a Quadrant 1, 2, or 3. Some will not. However, it will still make for a better organization.

Key Actions to Take with Quadrant 4 Physicians Include:

- Use the same actions as with Quadrants 1, 2, and 3 physicians.

- Resist the temptation to make believers out of these physicians. They represent only a small percentage of the medical staff.

FIGURE 8.2 | PHYSICIAN QUADRANT DESCRIPTIONS

LEVEL OF SUPPORT FOR CHANGE	DESCRIPTION	KEY ACTIONS
Quadrant 1 **"LOYAL"** *(Always)*	Physicians who are inherently supportive. They see the value in the changes the organization is making and will actively support those changes.	• Thank physicians for their support at a group or individual meeting. • Ask what the system does well. • Ask about and focus on key operational issues that if fixed would make their work better. • Send a note to all the departments complimented by the physicians, giving credit to the physicians for sharing this recognition.
Quadrant 2 **"Want to be aligned"** *(Usually)*	Physicians who want to be on board and are most of the time, but there is one thing that might be bothering them that keeps them from being fully aligned with system leaders. (e.g. an operational or political issue; frustration with a particular individual).	• Use the same actions as with Quadrant 1 physician. • If you cannot address a concern, say so and explain why. Physicians would rather hear a "no" than be left in limbo.
Quadrant 3 **"Skeptical"** *(Sometimes)*	Physicians who are skeptics that hang in the balance. These individuals have many issues and concerns. The organization will need to be relentless to move them, but they can be moved.	• Use the same actions as with Quadrant 1 and 2 physician. • Have frank discussions regarding operational issues that cannot be fixed at all or in the timeframe they would like. • Be especially persistent in capturing wins, as this group will have more concerns.
Quadrant 4 **"Naysayer"** *(Never)*	These physicians will most likely never be on board or move to Quadrant 1 or 2.	• Use the same actions as with Quadrant 1, 2 and 3 physician. • Resist the temptation to make believers out of these physicians. They only represent a small percentage of the medical staff.

115

Conducting Physician Quadrant Discussions

Below is an example of how the quadrant process works.

I recently conducted this exercise with about 16 senior leaders in an organization representing the flagship hospital, a smaller hospital, and the employed medical group of the system. The chief medical officers from different parts of the organization, the CEO and CFO of the system, the presidents of the hospitals in the system, the medical group president, and the other members of the senior team were at the session.

Before the meeting, the leaders were given the assignment to take a list of their physicians and, using the form provided (see Figure 8.3), identify and place each physician into one of the quadrants. Each of the leaders was asked to do this alone and without discussing their physician placements with each other.

Physician Name	Quadrants				Notes
	1	2	3	4	

FIGURE 8.3 | PHYSICIAN QUADRANT WORKSHEET

Everyone came to the meeting with their completed sheets, and some very real and honest discussions took place.

As the discussion began around the room, the chief medical officer said, "I think this physician is in Quadrant 2," and explained why. The president of the hospital this physician was affiliated with said, "I'd place her in Quadrant 3," and also explained why. Another attendee said, "My wife went to that physician and it was such a horrendous experience, I'm worried she won't even want to use any physicians in the place that I work."

After all this was said, they looked at each other and realized they had not been sharing their perception of the physicians with one another.

The discussion continued and another leader said, "I have a really good relationship with this physician. I don't know what happened that day, but that is not her usual behavior. This physician would want to know. I will meet with her to give her the feedback."

Then, another physician was placed in Quadrant 4. Someone said, "Why is he head of our service line if he's a Quadrant 4 physician?" The group then discussed the fact that they had given responsibility to an individual who was not aligned with the goals of the organization, thinking that this would align and change him. However, it did not.

In other words, there was a lot of very good discussion sparked by this exercise. By the end of the session, the topics of selection, feedback, and development needs were at the forefront of the leaders' minds.

What Does the Quadrant Exercise Accomplish for Your Organization?

The quadrant exercise has many positive benefits. For example:

1. All top leaders spend quality time discussing where each physician stands related to their alignment.

2. The exercise identifies potential and current physician leaders and champions.

3. It prioritizes the physicians' needs, which allows for specificity in follow-up.

4. It motivates leaders to work with physicians in their development.

5. It reduces burnout because it provides recognition, solicits input, demonstrates the organization's commitment to assisting physicians in feedback and development, and identifies operational improvements needed to create the optimal physician work environment.

Every organization we've worked with that has seen physician engagement go up near the top has learned how to maximize the Physician Quadrant tool. This tool, alongside rounding on physicians, makes up what I call the "chassis" that everything else can plug into. It is one of the foundation pieces for success in our efforts to engage physicians and alleviate burnout.

Day in the Life of a Physician

One other tool we've seen used very successfully is called "Day in the Life of a Physician." It's exactly what it sounds like. Each participating leader chooses a different physician to spend the entire day with. (It doesn't need to be the same day for every leader/physician pairing.)

This is meant to be a normal workday. If a physician is going to their clinic at a certain time, the leader will meet them there. Of course the leader needs to get permission to be present with patients, but patients are usually quite agreeable once the purpose is explained. Common sense needs to be used regarding when the leader shouldn't be in the room, but in general, they spend the day with the physician: outpatient clinic, inside the hospital, and any other setting.

Success has been achieved in helping organizations implement this tool. It's not uncommon for a leader to come back and say to us, "My gosh, I'm surprised they're not more frustrated than they are." But it has also helped fix some things that needed fixing. For example, after spending a day with the physician, a leader might say, "I think if we did this instead of that, it would be easier. We can make this change for the physician. I can see now why they want a printer over there because that's a pretty long walk."

A "Day in the Life of a Physician" has a number of advantages. One, it creates a relationship between the physician and the person shadowing them. Two, it demonstrates to the physician that we're interested in walking a mile in their shoes and that their input is welcomed. Three, it helps us reward and recognize things that are working well. Four, it leads to really, really excellent process improvement and quality improvement. And five, it gives the person who is shadowing empathy for the physician's life, which they will likely share with colleagues from then on.

This has been found to be an inexpensive way to improve efficiency and effectiveness in an organization. It's one of those cost-effective actions that leads to better operations and better relationships.

CHAPTER NINE:

ORGANIZATIONAL MEASUREMENT TOOLS

E veryone in healthcare understands how vital measurement is to tracking the health of an organization. The three tools described in this chapter—Provider Feedback System^{SM}, stoplight report, and administrative dashboard—all measure high-impact items. They help align goals, show progress toward meeting them, and create a better culture—specifically, the type of culture all stakeholders thrive in, including physicians.

Provider Feedback System^{SM}

As mentioned in Part 1, although physicians thrive on evidence and are data driven, research shows they do not receive data on patient care as often as one would think. This is ironic since physicians are actually one of the best audiences to present data to—after all, they are dedicated to finding out how they're doing and working to do better.

Physicians want to be our partners in improvement. To make that happen, sharing timely and relevant data with them consistently and seeking their feedback is key. One of the best tools I have seen for doing this and more is the Provider Feedback System. It's not only an engagement and alignment tool, but also a performance improvement and reward & recognition tool all in one.

This tool was created by Studer Group®. There are other feedback systems out there, but I find that many are so cumbersome that physicians are overwhelmed by the information they receive. The Provider Feedback System provides easy-to-understand metrics as well as summaries to help physicians see which metrics are the most important.

The Provider Feedback System creates a number of plusses for physicians. It helps them understand the strategic plan of the organization and where they fit in it. They mutually work with someone assigned by the healthcare system to review and decide which goals they most need to achieve and to rate the importance and priority of each goal.

So let's walk through this process from the beginning.

Step #1: Set Organizational Goals

The Provider Feedback System is much like the Studer Group Leader Evaluation Manager®, a tool created to provide feedback to leaders and to set weighted and clear objectives. Basically this tool was adjusted for physicians and other care providers.

For example, an organization might have one of their desired outcomes be to achieve a certain number of patient visits. To achieve this patient visit goal, each physician has a patient visit goal. When these goals are all added together, they should match the organizational goal.

Another goal might be around access. The organization's goal is to have patients able to see a primary care physician within so many days or even hours of when they call to get an appointment. For specialists, the goal might be around how long it takes to get the consult when a primary care physician refers patients to their specialty.

Step #2: Set Individual Goals, Rank Metrics, and Prioritize

First, we set each physician's goals. Try to limit these goals to no more than eight or so. There might be a goal for Patient Experience, a few goals under the area of Quality, a few goals under Finance, and certainly a goal in the area of Volume Growth. Certain physicians might also have a goal under People, specifically if they have high turnover in their practice or low employee engagement.

To be clear, leaders don't just "assign" these metrics to physicians. It's a partnership. The physician is provided with an overarching list of possible metrics, and the physician reviews them and picks what the key goals are they want to achieve.

Once goals have been set, the metrics come next. For example, the goal is set with a physician to get 90 percent of patients seen within 15 minutes of their appointment time. The recommended approach is to use a 5-point scale: Meeting the goal is a 3, exceeding the goal at an agreed-upon level is a 4, and greatly exceeding the goal is a 5. Going the other way, a 2 is underperforming, and a 1 is very much underperforming.

FIGURE 9.1 | 5 POINT SCALE EXAMPLE

Increase the percent of patients that saw provider within 15 minutes of appointment time from 85% to 90%

Metric	Description	Scale
5	Greatly Exceed the Goal	5 = above 95%
4	Exceed the Goal	4 = 93 – 94%
3	Meet the Goal	3 = 90 – 92%
2	Under-perform the Goal	2 = 85 – 89%
1	Greatly Under-perform the Goal	1 = less than 84%

Working together with the physician to set these goals allows for a far more effective individualized approach.

Then prioritization takes place. Weighting the goals helps to communicate with the individual physician what is most important for them to focus on. A typical rule of thumb for weighting of goals is as follows: A weight of 10 percent creates awareness, a weight of 20 percent creates focus, and a weight of 30 percent or more creates urgency.

For example, in an academic setting, a physician is responsible for teaching, meeting research/publishing deadlines, and oversight of patient visits/care. The physician might naturally tend to lean toward one or two of the responsibilities, but this weighting allows the organization and the physician to talk through and get clear on what is most important.

During all these sessions to set the goals for each physician, it will be natural for the physician to bring up operational improvements they feel are needed for them to achieve the goals. This is great. It assists administration in aligning their own and the organization's priorities. It creates the conversation that is paramount to relationship-building. Ultimately, it leads to achieving the desired outcomes while also creating a positive working relationship.

A good feedback system gives the physician a greater sense of control and input, a higher quality of performance, and an awareness of opportunities to improve. And, of course, physicians who are aligned and engaged will help the organization achieve its operational goals— thus its mission.

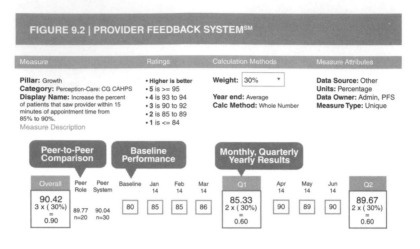

The Provider Feedback System leads to an evolution that aligns to the changing healthcare reimbursement environment and sets the stage for a shift in how physician compensation is formulated.

Stoplight Report

Another helpful tool is the stoplight report. It allows organizations to keep their "wins" at the forefront so that physicians and others can see and feel good about what has been accomplished. In working with many healthcare leaders, my experience has been that they are so busy moving to the next challenge that they don't get to enjoy the wins enough.

Working with a senior executive team not so long ago, they asked me what my number-one recommendation to them would be. I told them my number-one recommendation would be to learn how to maximize and optimize wins. One doesn't receive a win once and move on, but rather receives it over and over and over again by holding the gains.

The stoplight report enables this to happen. It's a simple yet powerful tool that organizations can use to show the status of suggestions physicians have offered and the action being taken.

The stoplight report is divided into three columns: Green = "Done"; Yellow = "In Progress"; and Red = "It Won't Happen."

Green means that a particular issue is resolved. For example, it could be that patient labs are now coming back in a certain time frame, or that a new phone system is installed, or that a piece of equipment was purchased and installed. When an organization leaves these "fixed" items on the stoplight report for a while, physicians will be able to say, "They have done a lot of things!" In fact, you can tell how good an organization is at fixing things by looking at the colors. If there is a lot of green, a good amount of yellow, and just a little bit of red, the organization is moving forward.

Yellow means the issue has been identified and that things are in progress. There's nothing wrong with having a lot of yellow on a report, as long as it's understood that the issues are going to move to green. Yellow means an issue has been identified and there is a focus to fix it. The physicians know it's on the administration's to-do list. They have been listened to and trust is increased.

The last part of the stoplight is red. There's nothing wrong with an item being in the red column. Sometimes the answer just has to be no. Physicians have told me that they'd rather hear a solid no than to feel they're just being glad-handed.

For example, I was recently in an organization whose physicians really wanted a new children's hospital. Unfortunately, building one would cost about $155 million. In talking to the CEO of the hospital, he said, "We can't build a new children's hospital. What we can do is redo part of our surgery recovery room and designate it for children." In a case like this one, the new children's hospital would be put in the "red" column for now. But the remodeled area for children to have a better recovery from surgery would go in the "yellow" column and move to "green" when the area is completed.

The challenge with the stoplight report is to keep it in front of everyone. Stoplights aren't hidden in the bushes. They're right out on the highway. That means that everybody on the executive team has to know what the stoplight report looks like. That means that it not only needs to be sent out to physicians but to everyone who has an impact on the physicians' work environment.

A few tips for using stoplight reports:

- Keep reports updated.
- Hang updated stoplight reports in physician lounges.

- Share them in all meetings in which attendees impact the physician work environment.

- Put some specifics from the stoplight report in the newsletter (or send them out as email blasts/updates).

- Recognize contributors who pointed out something that will benefit everyone. You can recognize them publicly and also send a personal thank-you note for input.

- Share with all department leaders. One may learn something from an idea in another area.

- Show connection of all and celebrate progress. (Example: Maintenance has solved 25 issues in Q1 based on input from our physicians.)

FIGURE 9.3 | STOPLIGHT REPORT

Department/Unit/Clinic:		Date:

COMPLETED (GREEN)	IN PROGRESS (YELLOW)	CAN'T COMPLETE AT THIS TIME & HERE'S WHY (RED)
AIDET℠ training for physicians is requested. Online training module was created and link sent to all medical staff as well as a 60-minute session will be presented at the medical staff meeting.	Sound barrier at Dr. G. nursing pods requested. (P. Little getting quotes)	Overhead storage cabinet for S. Hicks, FNP (Due to cost, this project cannot be completed at this time)
OB Doppler requested by Dr. S. was purchased and delivered.	Additional Ortho mid-level provider needed. (Recruitment has begun)	Peds physicians do not feel expansion to level 2 nursery was enough. (No capital resources at this time. Will target for consideration within 5 year strategic plan)
Dual Monitors purchased and installed for all providers.	Laser Equipment for pigmented skin and tattoo removal requested by Dr. B. (Will be considered in the next budget process that begins in October)	OB physicians requesting higher pay for PAs. (Conducted a salary and benefits compensation study and were found to be within competitive range -- no changes at this time and will be reviewed yearly)
On-line printer for LeAnn M.'s office ordered and installed for use on 1E.	More staffing in OR requested. (Continuing outreach and training of internal candidates. Expected to be fully staffed in less than one month)	
More chairs needed for physicians to sit when visiting patients in rooms. Provided one marked chair per room.	Training for new medication reconciliation feature in EPIC system is requested. (Training session by EPIC champions is in planning stages and training schedule will be announced in 2 weeks)	
Scribes requested in ED. 2 scribes were hired for pilot project.		
Pediatric Oximetry / Dual Monitors and standing station for Dr. H. installed.		
Lighted Curettes requested by R. Finch, FNP ordered and installed.		

Administrative Dashboard

Another technique to solicit input from physicians and create alignment is the administrative dashboard. At times, things come about during meetings with physicians that can create a knowledge gap between physicians and administration.

In my role as an administrator of a hospital, I sat in on executive medical staff meetings. On my way to a meeting one evening, I ran into the chairmen of one of the departments, who told me he felt the hospital was running better. As I walked into the meeting, I felt optimistic. I was ready. I was certain this was going to be a good executive medical staff meeting.

The meeting began with a welcome from the president of the medical staff, and then time was provided for each department to report to the group. When it was time for the report from the chairman with whom I had spoken, he led off with one or two things that the department was upset about. Next thing I knew, everybody was coming up with things they were upset about, one after another. This "positive meeting" that I thought was going to be a piece of cake turned out to be anything but that.

After the meeting, I went and talked to this physician and said, "I'm a little confused. Help me understand. On the way down the hall, you told me all these good things, yet in the meeting, you reported only what was wrong." He responded, "I have only so much time and we need to fix what's wrong."

I got it. I guess if you have only so much time, you're going to have to first focus on what needs fixing before talking about what's going better.

Another surprise I got that day was that one of the complaints was about one of the most well-run departments in the whole organization. Typically, we never heard a complaint about this area. On that day, though, what I heard was that we were way behind in medical re-cords. I was stunned. The next day I went to the Medical Records Department and shared with Pat, the leader of the department, the feedback I had received.

She said, "Oh yes, we are behind on medical records." She then went on to tell me that an employee's mother had gotten ill and she had taken off. Another one had a death in the family, so she was also gone. Yet another one had a pregnancy that had suddenly turned complicated and she had to go on bed rest. So this department had lost three staff members in less than 72 hours.

Now, obviously, these were unavoidable absences, and this leader was really competent. She already had a plan in place. She told me what her solution was and when the department would be caught up. Her response was really competent, and I had no complaints about it. My only wish was that I had had this information before the meeting.

This situation very much reminds me of an error in the media. So many people have already read the article, that when the correction eventually comes out, the misin-formation has already had wide circulation. Whether it's deserved or not, the damage is already done. So I started thinking of ways to get ahead of this kind of challenge in the future.

At the next executive medical staff meeting, I asked them to create a dashboard for me. I explained how we seem to always create dashboards for them, and it was timely for them to create a dashboard for me. I asked that this dashboard identify six, seven, eight, or a maximum of ten things in the organization that are the most vital to them. We had a good conversation and decided to carry the subject over to the next meeting.

We exchanged ideas back and forth over the next few weeks. Items placed on our dashboard included decreasing nursing turnover, moving patients through the hospital so they didn't sit in the Emergency Department for so long, getting lab reports back in a certain amount of time, and OR turnaround and start times. We all agreed that it was a good start.

An official administrative dashboard was created, and there were about seven departments that provided the data and the metrics that went on that dashboard. Next we decided what the goal was for each item. The department leaders provided what their results were prior to the medical staff meeting. It was decided that each month on the Monday before the meeting, the dashboard would be updated and come to me so that I could review and prepare.

I could look at the dashboard, and if we were a little behind on an item, I could learn more to provide an explanation. Then at meetings when I gave the administrative report, we covered the dashboard. I could bring up, "As you can see, we're behind in lab reports. Here's what we're doing to fix it." The wins were also reviewed.

The dashboard also let the physicians see how often certain things happen. I remember one day sitting in a meeting knowing that a physician was ready to bring up an issue. However, after he read the metrics, he realized it was an isolated experience. Do I wish it didn't happen?

Absolutely. But being able to see that it was an isolated experience helped him keep it in perspective.

What did creating this administrative dashboard accomplish? First of all, it helped the physicians because they now felt they had input into making the organization more efficient and effective and determining the desired outcomes. This helps alleviate the feeling of loss of control that so often contributes to physician burnout. It also helps physicians feel appreciated, which goes a long way toward helping them get engaged and aligned and stay that way.

CHAPTER TEN:

ORGANIZATIONAL TREATMENT TOOLS

With the diagnostic work complete and with the measurement strategy in place, it is time to look at various tools and tactics that create the positive work environment for physicians that will help prevent and heal physician burnout.

The seven tools described in this section—physician selection/retention; rounding on physicians; focus, fix, and follow-up; reward and recognition; patient call backs; physician preference cards; and simulation labs—address key items that are vital to an organization. Choose the tools and techniques that best match up with your particular needs and situation.

This approach is similar to a football team that has some basic plays that they normally run, but depending on what happens, they can make adjustments. They're still running the basic formations, however. In healthcare, standardization creates excellence.

Physician Selection and Retention

As discussed, physicians desire input and a feeling of control over their environment, as well as the knowledge that things are being run efficiently and effectively and that patients are receiving quality care. When these needs are met, it has a positive impact on physician burnout. One big satisfier on all these fronts is making sure physicians have input into who will be part of the organization.

It's important to be careful that one stays close to what made physician selection so successful in years past. When studying peer interviews in the early 1990s, we learned a lot from physician groups. If a group had three oncologists and they were bringing in a fourth one, everyone made sure they knew that physician. In fact, it was very unlikely for a physician to be hired who did not meet with every physician in the group.

Most of the groups were very small. If a group was larger and a candidate couldn't meet every physician in the group, they'd meet everyone in their area of specialty. Whether it was pediatrics, radiology, surgery, general surgery, etc., the candidate would know everyone by the time they were hired.

Today, it is not always feasible for a potential hire to meet everyone. That's just the reality in our age of new employment structures and larger, more integrated health systems. However, it is possible to give many physicians the chance to have input into the selection process.

Preparing for the Interview

When starting to interview physicians, it's easy to feel that a solid interview system is in place. But even if you do, it is important to go back to all physicians in the group and say, "Your input is needed. Here are the specific job descriptions we have built. Here are the specific qualities that are being looked for in this physician. Here's the type of training we're looking for. Here's the type of experience we're looking for. Do you agree? Disagree? Can you tell us why?" So you include the physician in creating the matrix used to assess the interviewee. (See Figure 10.1)

This is a very important step, because creating the matrix provides the physicians with more control over who's going to get selected. The input provided will also likely yield the best candidate. If physician input is not gathered, issues will come up later. Also, if the candidate doesn't meet all of the requirements, this needs to be communicated back along with the reasoning behind the decision. For example, the physicians might say that a physician with 15 years' experience is needed. That means if we're recruiting someone who doesn't have 15 years' experience, it will be important to go back and explain why the person we hire is a good fit. In other words, even if we end up not recruiting the person physicians are advocating for, they will still have inclusion and input into the process.

FIGURE 10.1 | SAMPLE MATRIX

Candidate _____
Position _____
Interviewer _____
Date _____

Core Competency Question (Tell me about a time when you...)	Score 1-5	Comments/Notes
1. TEAMWORK AND COLLABORATION		
2. CARING AND COMPASSION		
3. COMMUNICATION		
4. LEADERSHIP		
5. JUDGMENT AND PROBLEM SOLVING		
6. VALUE YOU WOULD BRING TO US		
TOTAL		
AVERAGE SCORE		

1:	2:	3:	4:	5:
•No experience	•Limited experience	•Specific experience	•Strong experience	•In-depth experience
•No cited examples	•Few examples cited	•Specific cited examples	•Strong cited examples	and ability to teach others
•Skills not evident	•Limited skills	•Evident skills	•Solid skills	•Exemplary cited examples
				•In-depth skills

Additional Comments:

Recommend [ ]   Do Not Recommend [ ]

The Interview

Next comes peer interviewing. This tactic has been used for years with physicians. Now that so many physicians are part of a larger whole, not all members of a group can be involved in selection, particularly if they have a different specialty from the new hire. At a minimum, consider having all physicians vet the questions that are to be asked during the interview and that are placed in the interview matrix. This allows all physicians to be familiar with the process, and it also provides that crucial feeling of input.

Physicians chosen for the interviewing team are those who have been identified as high-performing contributors to the medical group and who model the standards of the group in attitude and behavior as well as in clinical competence. They are physicians who are willing to participate in training in the selection process, have a clear understanding of the job responsibilities, and who communicate well and have strong listening skills.

The selection team, consisting of current physicians, chooses who will ask which questions to the candidate and who will dig deeper into certain areas. They also select who will be involved in deeper reference checks if needed, and they decide which physician will cover topics of most interest to the candidate and their family—such as housing, schools, and so forth.

While the organization's head of physician recruitment is usually excellent with these kinds of "community" details, having a physician cover them means a great deal to the candidate and their family. It also creates a deeper bond between the organization and the recruited physicians and their families. Remember, decisions such as these are still made as much with the heart as with the mind.

Onboarding

When the time comes to onboard a physician, assigning a "buddy" helps. This is evident in our work with other clinical areas. However, in many organizations the "buddy system" is not used with physicians. In my opinion this is a missed opportunity. Why not assign a physician a mentor or a mentee during the onboarding process?

In working with a medical group, the physician engagement survey showed one of the notable disappointments identified by some of the new physicians was, "I came here because in the interview process I met Dr. X and I was looking forward to working with her. Now that I'm here, though, I hardly ever see her."

Particularly for young physicians, it can be disappointing to feel that "I am on my own." Even if a new physician doesn't get to work with a physician who recruited them, it is important to make sure that they still have mentors, preceptors, and people that they can go to.

Follow-up

The Studer Group® books *Practicing Excellence* and *Engaging Physicians* discuss the importance of follow-up with physicians. It really is critical to circle back with physicians and make sure that everything is going well.

For non-physicians, research shows us that the first 90 days of employment are critical. Thus, a 30- and 90-day meeting/checkup with each new employee is conducted. (See my book *Hardwiring Excellence*, pages 173-179, to learn more.)

With physicians, it's a different situation, and a longer timeframe is needed. Instead, three- and six-month meetings are recommended. These meetings are focused on specific questions. For instance: *How well do we compare to what we said we're going to be? What's really going well at your practice? What do you feel good about? What are some areas that you are concerned about, that you feel could be improved upon? What are some ideas you have to improve the work environment here, improve patient care, and so on? Is there anyone here that you would like us to reward and recognize?*

Here are some of the things that are accomplished with the three- and six-month checkups:

- The physician knows the organization is interested in their viewpoint. (input)

- The organization learns ways to improve onboarding if something has been missed. (input/ quality and efficiency)

- The questions focus the conversation around the positive aspects of the new employment situation as opposed to focusing solely on the challenges that any new staff member experiences. (appreciation)

- Names of people who have been helpful are gathered and can be followed up with. (appreciation)

- Any issues are identified and can be addressed, which leads to better care. (quality and efficiency)

By creating a world-class selection and onboarding process, an organization reduces physician burnout as well as making any needed improvements.

Rounding on Physicians

Not too long ago, another group of healthcare professionals was feeling burned out. Into the mid-1990s, it was hard to recruit a nurse—despite the presence of nurse recruiters, an attractive and welcoming website, a cadre of gifts, and so forth. Besides searching the website, nurses would talk to other individuals who worked at an organization, and often those conversations would lead to the nurse's (unfavorable) decision.

Fortunately our industry was able to make some needed changes, and before long nursing again became a sought-after profession. But that's not the point here. The point is that just as the biggest driver of where patients go is word of mouth, the same is true of professionals. A nurse talks to another nurse. And a physician talks to another physician. Organizations need to leverage this truth.

Years ago, I was in a city that was experiencing a nursing shortage. The organization had planned a big nurse recruitment fair. However, they had not invited the nurses already working at the organization to the event. When

I heard this, I suggested that they either quickly expand the invitation to all the nursing staff or consider canceling the event. Romancing a group of nurses not even working for the organization while ignoring the nurses already employed might hurt them in the long-run.

Apply the same principle to physicians.

I was working with an organization whose physician engagement hovered around the 50th percentile—not really bad or really good. With that outcome, the organization had about a 50/50 shot that when a recruited physician called a current physician to find out about the work environment, they would hear, "Yeah this is a great place. Come work for us." So, this organization decided to focus on one strategy at a time to help move these results. Their starting point? Rounding for outcomes.

Studer Group has covered rounding to some degree in all of our books, as it is truly a key to engaging all staff members. And rounding is a foundational and integral step to providing physicians with a good place to provide care.

Who Should Round?

A common question is "Who should round on the physician?" The answer varies. If you're an academic medical center, it's certainly the department chair. If it's a community hospital, various physician leaders should round. There is also nothing wrong with having non-physician leaders round on a physician. What matters is that whoever rounds has the skill to do it well and is able to execute on the follow-up of the feedback received.

Effective Rounding

Rounding for outcomes with the physician is a method of creating and building a relationship, but it's also more than that. It's about having a relationship that leads to higher levels of physician engagement as well as better clinical and organizational outcomes.

There are at least four things to cover in rounding on a physician.

FIGURE 10.2 | ROUNDING ON PHYSICIANS	
1	Make a human and personal connection.
2	Ask, "What is working well today?"
3	Ask, "Do you have everything you need to provide excellent care to your patient today?"
4	Ask, "Anybody to reward and recognize?"

1. Make a human and personal connection. The number-one step is making a human connection. For example, when I rounded on Dr. Sidney Clements, I asked about his children, because he is a dad, and talked about baseball because I know he is a huge baseball fan. When I rounded on Dr. Bob Frank, I asked about his two daughters and their plans for high school and college.

2. Ask, "What is working well?" Next ask, "What is working well?" In healthcare, people are naturally tuned to looking at what's going wrong. Physicians in particular are trained to look for disease and abnormalities. Rounding is a good way to keep the positive alive—if a proactive effort is not made, it just isn't done.

3. Ask, "Do you have everything you need to provide excellent care to your patients today?" Ask physicians about how easy it is to practice medicine at your organization. Do they have everything they need to take excellent care of their patients? This is really what physicians look for in any organization, because it connects to the ability to take the best possible care of the patient, so it is a critical question to ask. At this point, the physician is either going to answer yes or no.

- If the answer to this question is no, and there is something the physician is concerned about, don't assume nothing has gone well. But also, don't miss this chance to dig a little deeper into what went wrong and what needs to go better. Here is your chance to focus on it, talk about it, document it, and follow up on it. (Focus, fix, and follow-up, which is our next physician must-have, will be addressed a bit later.)

- If they say yes, things are great, dig deeper and ask for specifics such as what is going well and why things went right. This answer moves us naturally to harvesting names for reward and recognition.

4. Ask, "Anybody to reward and recognize?" Rounding provides an opportunity for leaders to collect and pass along recognition to physicians and staff who have been helpful. What gets recognized gets repeated, so when individuals are thanked for specific behaviors, they are more likely to repeat the behaviors.

How Often Should I Round?

Now that how to effectively round has been discussed, let's talk about how often to round. There is no single answer. Every organization functions differently. The answer also depends on the role of the physicians being rounded on as well as their impact (for example, maybe someone brings in a high percentage of patient volume). However, as a general rule, the more often you can round on physicians, the better.

It is found that if physicians are rounded on once a month using the prescribed model of rounding, physician engagement will be in the top 15 percent (and many times in the top 10 percent). If physicians are rounded on once a quarter, physician engagement will be in the top 25 percent. If physicians are rounded on every six months or only once a year or never, their engagement is pretty much 50 percent or lower.

The message is that if there is to be a positive impact on physician engagement, an organization should plan to round on physicians at least quarterly and in some cases monthly.

Rounding tips:

- Start somewhere. Make a plan on your schedule to round on a certain number of physicians per week. This is as important as any other meeting and will help you be proactive to their needs instead of reactive.

- Keep rounding conversations to the point.

Focus, Fix, and Follow-up

This tactic can be used in conjunction with rounding or as a standalone. It ties into the concept of input, efficiency, quality, and appreciation.

For physicians, a key issue is the feeling of losing control. Physicians think, *I want quality of care for my patients. I want efficient, effective operations. I want input, and it wouldn't be bad to be appreciated, either.* While all tactics hit one or more of these drivers, focus, fix, and follow-up hits all four of them solidly.

FIGURE 10.3 | FOCUS, FIX, AND FOLLOW-UP		
FOCUS:	*Focus on what the physician is saying.*	▶ Input
FIX:	*Fix it so the physician can have more efficient / effective operations and better quality of care for the patients.*	▶ Quality ▶ Efficiency
FOLLOW-UP	*Follow-up so the physician is communicated with and is appreciated for identifying the issue.*	▶ Appreciation

In most physician engagement surveys, one of the top dissatisfiers is around administrative responsiveness. Focus, fix, and follow-up was developed with an eye on responsiveness, but it also accomplished many other things.

Focus

When asking a physician questions, talking to a physician, or getting information in some manner from a physician (it could be in written form), identify and focus on the issue raised during the rounding process. When focus is placed on a particular issue, the scope is narrowed to a manageable level. High performance is narrowing the scope of the issue and then sequencing the tactics, strategies, or behaviors to fix the issue.

A physician might say, "One of the problems is that the ORs are running late." So, focus on the issue at hand. Ask specific questions that dig deeper into why the OR is running late, how this affects the physician, solutions they might have to help fix the problem, etc.

Fix

From data collection to a change of procedures, fix the issue. Train staff, improve processes, or buy a new piece of equipment. Keep the physician up-to-date as the process unfolds. It is vital to let the physician know each step of the way. If it cannot be fixed, say so and explain why.

Follow-up

Make sure to validate the focus, fix, and follow-up data and communicate it out into the organization. There are a variety of ways to do this. Make sure that every time focus, fix, and follow-up is used, data is collected and the information is communicated out into the organization. Update each item at medical exec meetings, talk about the activity in the medical group meetings, and discuss each item at the service line meetings. And so on.

Imagine, for example, that a physician complains about the number of hospital-acquired pressure ulcers. An organization intent on earning physician loyalty might first review the data to determine if it is indeed a widespread problem. If so, the organization could ask physicians to participate in teaching modules and then keep a scoreboard in nursing lounges so everyone could measure progress in reducing pressure ulcers. However, many leaders forget one of the most important parts of the process: to follow up and capture the win! Once pressure ulcers have dropped and remained low, continue to communicate these results to physicians.

Reward and Recognition

Physicians go through more change than probably any other category of healthcare professional. The amount of reading they have to do to keep up with the research is absolutely phenomenal. The number of new medications, new techniques, and new tools that are introduced to physicians would be overwhelming to most of us.

It is easy to think that because of the nature of a physician's work that they don't need reward and recognition. It's easy to think their value and the impact they have on others goes without saying. However, this is not true. Don't underestimate the importance of reward and recognition to a physician.

No matter what your employment status is, no matter where you are or what you do, when you work in healthcare, you are a part of "the great patient care team" and deserve to be recognized for your contributions. This includes key stakeholders in your organization, employees, volunteers, patients and their families—and yes, physicians.

Thank-You Notes

Thank-you notes, especially sent to physicians' homes, have great impact. In a study of the top workplace incentives, the number-one strategy was handwritten thank-you notes.[1]

There's nothing difficult about the act of writing a thank-you note, but there are proven ways to make them more effective for physicians and to hardwire them in your organization.

Ask each nurse leader, unit nurse, or other managers in the organization to send one handwritten thank-you note to a physician's home on a regular basis. Harvesting "wins" and recognition for specific physicians from their daily rounding with employees should provide leaders with the information needed to send a personal "thank you" to physicians. Physicians who receive such a note typically seek out the person who sent it, so the good feelings generated by these interactions go in both directions.

It's also important to tell the CEO who is being thanked and why so they can extend their appreciation the next time they see the physician, or write a thank-you note to them as well. A thank-you note from the CEO or another senior leader for specific actions or outcomes is also powerful. In addition to delighting the physicians and strengthening their connection with the person who wrote the note, the specific behaviors mentioned in the note will be reinforced.

Organizations that send thank-you notes consistently have created some type of system, such as a grid, to help make this skill a habit. To create this grid, list the names of key physicians in one column. Start with those who you believe are "loyal" in regard to their level of support for change. Add additional columns for each week or month over the next year and then simply check off the boxes as you send thank-you notes to your key physicians.

Further, organizations may choose to encourage physicians with high levels of loyalty and engagement with the organization to send thank-you notes to nurses and other staff as a mechanism to foster positive relationships between all parties.

Spotlight Physicians

Mention specific physicians who are making a difference whenever you can. This is especially effective at board meetings. Start the meeting with recognition of a physician. For example, the CEO might say, "Dr. Ross came in during a day off to work with the OR team to update surgical preference cards for physicians. This has increased efficiency and reduced costs. As the board chair, I recommend the board write a letter of appreciation to Dr. Ross."

An organization in which we worked in Massachusetts wanted to do something special for Doctors' Day. They asked everybody in the organization to write a note or a paragraph about a physician and the difference that physician made in a person's life—whether that person was an employee, a patient, or a family member. So the employees started writing, and the notes were placed on a long wall of the hospital. All of a sudden, a feeding frenzy began. Physicians were swarming down the hallway and crowding around to read these notes that people had written about them.

Some individuals had written notes about their personal experience with the physician as a patient or family member. Others had written expressions of appreciation for how the physician would take time to teach them. Some told stories about unspoken acts of kindness or sacrifices that they had seen the physician do for a patient or family.

I remember one of the stories was about a young child who was really ill and he really had a taste for a certain milkshake from a certain restaurant. The physician left and came back later with the milkshake the child was craving.

This idea caught on throughout the hospital, and before long, the hallway was loaded with tributes to physicians. The physicians whose names were mentioned felt very good. However, another unexpected thing happened when some of the physicians noticed their names weren't there. Those physicians must have thought, *What do I have to do to get my name there, too?* because all of a sudden their behavior started adjusting. In other words, the wall of physician praise was a feel-good event, but it didn't end there.

In fact, the physicians loved it so much that they decided to write notes about what nursing means to them for Nurses Week. Some wrote paragraphs about nursing in general, while others wrote about individual units or individual nurses. They hung these notes again in the hallway. This time, staff and physicians were stopping to read these notes—heartwarming proof of the great teamwork and positive things that were happening in the hospital.

Don't underestimate the importance of appreciation to a physician. It makes a difference and, as this story illustrates, can have an amazing ripple effect throughout the organization.

Patient Call Backs

The next tactic is post-visit calls made to patients. These calls can be made by nurses, call centers, and even by physicians themselves. While these calls are intended to assure quality care and follow-up, they also provide a valuable method to receive positive feedback for physicians.

I just saw some reports from one of Studer Group's coaches and they showed that once the organization put in the patient call-back system, not only did its care improve, but so did recognition of physicians. To understand why, let's walk through the typical call:

When a patient leaves a healthcare system or an out-patient clinic, they receive a post-care call. The caller expresses empathy and concern up front. And here's a suggestion to make the call even more impactful. The patient knows they came for a test because the physician ordered it, right? Try saying, "Your physician wanted us to call." For example: "Miss Stanzell, this is Nurse Betsy from AZ Clinic. Dr. Hollis wanted to make sure that I gave you a call today to talk about where things are going."

All of a sudden, the call to the patient is made because the physician asked for it to be made. That knocks their socks off. Some physicians do this already—particularly surgeons—and there's a good reason for it. When you make the call and you frame it correctly, everybody wins.

The caller then asks about medication, understanding of post-visit instructions, and follow-up appointments. So, during the call, often the clinical items are covered early on. The key is to lead with the questions concerning their care, making sure the clinical outcomes are dealt with, and then to move into questions relating to the patient experience.

FIGURE 10.4	SAMPLE PATIENT CALL BACK	
Empathy and Concern	Hello Mrs. Smith. This is Mike from the Cardiology Clinic. Dr. Jones asked that I call and check on you after your recent visit to our facility. Is this a good time?
Clinical Outcomes	• Were your discharge instructions clear and understandable? Please tell me in your own words how you are to care for yourself at home. • Are you having any unusual symptoms or problems? (Specific to problem- i.e. dressing, PAIN, bruising or swelling, N/V; e.g., Do your favorite pair of shoes still fit?) • Have you filled your new prescriptions yet? Do you have any questions about those medications? • Were you able to make a follow-up appointment with the physician?
Reward and Recognition	Are there any physicians, nurses or staff that you would like us to recognize for doing an excellent job?
Process Improvement	Thank you for taking the time to share with me about your care and recovery. Do you have any suggestions for us?

Also key is harvesting reward and recognition as appropriate through the call. Ask, "We like to reward and recognize people here. Is there anybody you'd like us to reward and recognize? Any departments you'd like to recognize?"

If they say something was spectacular, dig in a little if possible. After all, it is known what room they were in and when their admission and discharge dates were. In an outpatient clinic, it is known what day they came in for a test or procedure. So if the patient says someone did an outstanding job and they're unaware of the name, collect the department and the name. This allows us to send the recognition back to the right person.

One of the questions to ask is this: "We have an excellent medical staff. Are there any physicians you would like us to reward and recognize or compliment? Would you like to give them your thank you?" This creates an opportunity for the patient to provide the names of a number of physicians.

So collect a lot of positive information on physicians. Now when rounding on physicians, and when it comes time to do other forms of reward and recognition, a "positive bank account" is established and can be drawn from if needed at a later time.

Finally, of course, harvest opportunities for process improvement.

So what does the post-visit call accomplish in terms of physician engagement? First, it positions the physician in a positive light. It certainly provides a better quality of care for the patient, which is one of the things that physicians are looking for. It provides improved efficiency and effectiveness because we're making sure we're capturing things we need to do better. If it is heard that there are some things that we can do better, they are captured, which can lead into focus, fix, and follow-up. And of course it provides many opportunities to reward and recognize physicians.

Like most of these tactics, organizations can customize the calls in a way that makes the most sense for them.

Physician Preference Cards

The goal of a golfer is to hit the ball with the club's "sweet spot." This creates a better shot with less effort. When playing baseball and the batter hits the ball with the sweet spot of the bat, once again the ball goes a lot farther and harder. So if two batters have the exact same swing, the one who hits on the sweet spot will have more success than the one who doesn't.

A similar principle holds true when an organization is creating a better work environment for physicians. When the physician's "sweet spot" is found, success follows. So, how is a person's sweet spot identified? Well, return once again to our list of physician drivers: that feeling of being in control, the ability to provide quality care for their patients, the efficiency and effectiveness of a system's operations, and a sense of appreciation. Those things that help the physician work at their optimal level of performance together make up the sweet spot.

With this in mind, let's talk about physician preference cards. Most people in healthcare are familiar with preference cards for surgeons. Why not create preference cards for all physicians? It not only makes things better for the physician, but for all staff who interact with the physician. Here is an example.

When is the first time a new nurse typically learns about a physician preference? Usually on their first night shift, when they wake a physician at 3 a.m. without all the information the physician needs to make a sound decision for a patient. We all know what happens. The nurse is brand new, probably hasn't really even met the physician, and certainly hasn't worked regularly with the physician to know what they might prefer when they receive a call.

So the physician answers the call and for whatever reason—perhaps this is the fifth call that night, or they have just received bad news on a patient, or they have their own sick child or something else is going on—the conversation may not be the kind that leads to building a strong relationship. The nurse is left with a bad feeling about the physician, and the physician is frustrated that perhaps the new nurses aren't trained as well as they need to be.

Physician preference cards help to change these kinds of scenarios and to facilitate a positive work culture. This tool provides a proactive way for nurses and others to learn how each physician works best. Physicians appreciate others knowing their preferences, employees appreciate being able to work more efficiently (and form more harmonious relationships with physicians), and patients appreciate the aligned coordination of their care.

Let's look at how this tool benefits surgeons. In a typical organization, before surgeons ever do a procedure, it is known what they need to make the operation highly successful, from scheduling to instrument placement and availability. We might even know their favorite music to play during surgery. In short, their preferences are known so the tools and equipment they need to do their job are provided.

But what about other non-surgeons, or even surgeons whose patients are out of surgery and in the units? Do we ask these practitioners about their preferences? If not, why not? If a preference card helps improve clinical outcomes, helps improve operations, and helps standardize processes and procedures, why wouldn't we use them for all physicians?

Think about a physician office staff sitting down with one of their physicians and saying, "We want this office to run really well. Tell us what you need to make that happen. What are your preferences?" That physician then might say, "Here's how I'd like the procedure trays to be prepared before I come to the room. I would like for you to round on my patients who are waiting more than 15 minutes for me. Here are the metrics I would like collected. This is how I want scheduling to take place. This is how I would like payment explained to the patient."

How Physician Preference Cards Work

Physician preference cards typically capture the physician's contact information, the time the physician rounds, information preferred prior to rounding, support requests, and other preferences. So, for example, if a nurse knows that a physician rounds between 7 and 8 a.m., they can ensure that their patient isn't being bathed during that hour and that current lab results are on the chart for the physician to review. As a result, physicians make fewer unnecessary trips to the hospital. Also, when nurses call, they have all the information the physician wants at their fingertips.

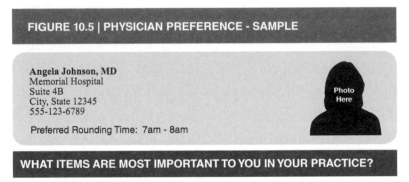

FIGURE 10.5 | PHYSICIAN PREFERENCE - SAMPLE

Angela Johnson, MD
Memorial Hospital
Suite 4B
City, State 12345
555-123-6789

Preferred Rounding Time: 7am - 8am

Photo Here

WHAT ITEMS ARE MOST IMPORTANT TO YOU IN YOUR PRACTICE?

1. Room and round on my patients that are delayed 15 minutes or more.

2. Make sure patient call backs are prioritized with a priority alert in my email.

3. Prep and open up minor procedure trays at time the patient is roomed.

4. Ensure the individualized patient care card which outlines the key care needs of the visit are completed prior to when I enter room for patient visit.

Rolling Out Physician Preference Cards

Begin by selecting physicians with whom you will pilot the tool. Factors to consider include physicians' responsiveness to new initiatives, nursing unit relationships with physicians, and other initiatives that may be taking place on nursing units at the same time. Choose the goals you will measure. Then determine what information you will collect to create the tool.

You might ask the physicians: "What three items are most important to you in your practice?" and/or "What is one item you would like to have improved?" Once you have interviewed physicians to collect the data and have implemented a preference card system, begin to solicit feedback from physicians on how well it is working.

Throughout the process, communicate extensively. Before the pilot, communicate to explain to staff and physicians why you are piloting the tool. During the feedback phase, send monthly updates to senior leaders, staff, and physicians. Capture the wins by sharing positive physician comments frequently and publicly. After a three-month pilot, review feedback and results with senior leadership to make a decision whether to expand the use of the tool.

Knowing physicians' preferences also helps the staff. This has been done for surgeons for years, and, ironically, I've never had surgeons or staff members say, "The preference card messed up our surgeries," or, "The preference card made it too individualized." In fact, a good leader can sit down with the surgery team and surgeons and explain that if the preference cards are used well, it helps to start more cases on time, and overall it will make their life better.

It's an interesting paradox. When individualizing physician preferences is started, it often leads to standardization of practice. You might say that's crazy. What I've learned is sometimes you have to do the behavior. When you do the behavior, you get the results. When you get results, you get the understanding of the physicians and the staff.

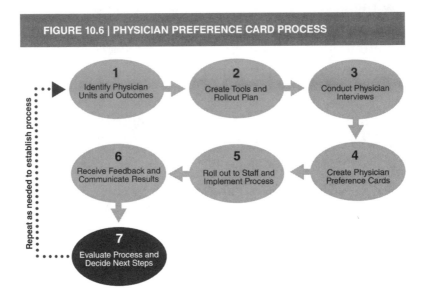

FIGURE 10.6 | PHYSICIAN PREFERENCE CARD PROCESS

The physician preference card hits all of the physician driver categories. The physician now gets to have input over what happens with patients and gains more control. Efficiency also improves. That input and that efficiency together improve quality of patient care. The physician feels appreciated.

Simulation Labs

Another tactic that is found to be helpful in providing a better work environment is conducting simulation labs with physicians. The lab is set so all the people who interact with a patient come into a room. Everybody role plays what they say and what they do. Then the rest of the staff give them feedback.

This was one of the ways that have been developed to practice tactics like key words at key times as care providers learn how to explain the side effects of medication. In healthcare, when people see it in action, rather than just hearing about it, they have a much better chance of doing it. That's why on the Studer website a learning lab is created and available where people can go in and actually see what right looks like.

Recently this tactic was modified for physicians. This process isn't easy, but I think it's worthwhile and it doesn't have to be that time-consuming. So how it worked was that a physician gathered together everybody who touches the patient—from the registration person to the certified nurse assistant to the nurse to the physician assistant or nurse practitioner—to walk through a simulated patient experience.

The "patient" was actually a person pretending to be a patient. She sat in a room. She didn't have to go to every entry point. And we said, "Okay, this person walks up to registration, she walks through exactly what you say and what you do and what you fill out." In this case, it all happened right on site, which was good because the patient was able to notice that if the registration person turned the computer screen a certain way, there would be better eye contact.

As they walked through the simulation, the physician told me how valuable it was. It gave him a much better understanding of everything the patient went through before she got to the physician. Sometimes, things were being done that staff members thought the physician wanted done that actually weren't all that necessary. It really helped the physician gain a better understanding of what everyone did, and it also led to process improvement.

It also really let the staff know what the physician was doing, which again led to better understanding and process improvement. It also led to some behavior changes regarding attitude or skill-building. The physician gave the viewpoint of "I'm going to say this here. So when the physician gets to the exam room, why don't you say it this way?" Then somebody else was able to say, "Why don't you explain it like this?" What it led to was everybody truly understanding the patient flow, allowing process improvement in the patient flow, and willingly and enthusiastically building skill sets.

Doing these skills labs does mean that you have to take a little bit of time to get everybody together, so, yes, you're going to lose some time. However, what I've learned over the years is that if you can get everyone together, you're going to lose a little bit of time up front, but you'll gain a lot of time for the rest of your career. The results more than make up for taking people out of their normal activities for a short amount of time to learn what the full process really is, how it works, and what everybody says and does.

People are in the habit of explaining what they do, so whoever facilitates a skills lab has to continue to remind them, "No, I don't want you explaining what you do; I want you to actually do it as if there's a patient there." While it may seem awkward at first, it will lead to a much better learning experience.

Skills labs may vary in size. In an effort to help physicians improve their communication skills and learn from peers, perhaps create a skills lab with at least three physicians—certainly no more than five at once. Three is best, and labs should take about 30 minutes. Each physician takes a turn at being the patient, the practicing physician, and the evaluator. After each turn, the patient and evaluator provide feedback about what the physician did particularly well, what they did or said to reduce anxiety, and what they did or said that may have increased it. At the end, each participant articulates two things they will do differently to better communicate with their patients.

Physicians *always* learn from each other and feel aligned to go forward and try something new—even if it's just a tweak to how they do things now. I typically facilitate to ensure good dialog and solid takeaways. The lab gives physicians an environment to practice what might feel awkward to them (for example, sitting down at a patient bedside or managing up the team). It also provides a rare opportunity to see what your peers do and together to commit to taking communication to the next level.

Like the other tools and tactics in this section, the skills lab impacts all the physician drivers. It gives physicians input into how they want to work with patients. It improves efficiency and effectiveness of patient visits (and thus, improves quality).

CHAPTER ELEVEN:

"OUT-OF-THE-BOX" TOOLS AND TACTICS

When one thinks of change, it is often thought of in terms of incremental change, which is good. Health systems take tactics that are already in operation and modify them, making gradual tweaks and improvements over time. This is a valuable and necessary method of change as it allows people to adjust their behavior at a sustainable pace so as not to be overwhelmed. As Aesop's fable "The Tortoise and the Hare" teaches: *Slow and steady wins the race.*

However, sometimes slow and steady change will not achieve the goal in the desired timeframe. At times a dramatic paradigm shift is called for. That's what this chapter is about. Its tactics are examples of "out-of-the-box" thinking organizations can adopt to help physicians avoid and cope with burnout.

It is time to recapture physicians. If our best and brightest are not won over now, the next generation will not be attracted to the medical field.

Physician Health and Wellness

Let's look at some other professions and what they provide "top-of-the-top" professionals. I know in health-care there are advantages to everybody being treated the same way. I get that. We're all on the same team. Nobody is better than anybody else. But the reality is that in roles, compensation, benefits, and in responsibility, there are differences. This is known to all.

When one thinks about physicians, their education, their training, their responsibility, their skin in the game, their need to stay up-to-date with research—their performance is really quite remarkable. They are the "top of the top" in our field, the super stars, and the elite professionals. You might think of them as the Navy SEALs, the Blue Angels, or even the modern-day Shakespeares, Beethovens, and Einsteins of our industry.

Let's review how other professions treat their "top-of-the-game" people to make sure they develop and keep performing at the highest possible level. After all, if we're depending on someone to save the lives of our patients, they need to be treated very, very well. The whole organization's future rests on physicians.

What other kinds of organizations have individuals who carry such weight? It's really quite remarkable how dependent we all are on physicians in a variety of ways.

My wife and I own a minor league baseball team with Bubba Watson, the professional golfer. The team is called the Pensacola Blue Wahoos, and they're based in Pensacola, FL. On the Pensacola Blue Wahoos, which is a Double-A team, there is a player named Jesse Winker. I like Jesse, for a number of reasons. One, he's just a fun guy when you get to know him. Two, he looks like my son-in-law, and I'm very fond of my son-in-law. Jesse Winker was drafted out of high school in what they call a supplemental round, which is an extended first round. That year the Reds signed him to a contract. They placed him in rookie ball, he moved on up, and now he's in Double-A ball.

Statistics show that when a player gets signed, there's a very small chance he'll ever play in the major leagues. However, major league teams invest heavily in all their players in the minor leagues. Jesse will play about 130 Double-A games with each game lasting about 2 hours and 45 minutes. Jesse might have six balls hit to him during a game, and he will be at bat about four times per game. You have to admit that in the grand scheme of things, this is not a ton of playing time. Yet, despite that, the Reds take very good care of Jesse.

For example, Jesse will be provided an organizational psychologist to work with him on how to position success and how to handle stress and failure. As major league baseball manager Buck Showalter says, the toughest distance for a baseball player is that six inches between the ears. They have to handle a lot of stress. A lot of people are counting on them. And they have to be able to handle failure, too. You see, if Jesse is an all-star, he'll hit 300. That means he'll make an out 70 percent of the time. When you are a baseball player and you make an out, it's devastating and you feel terrible. You've let the team down. You've let your organization down, and you have to go back in the dugout. And if it's the last out of the game, you feel even worse.

Jesse will also get a physical trainer and a strength and conditioning coach to make sure his body is working at its highest potential. He will have a nutritionist to help him learn how to eat right. But that's not all. He'll also have a hitting coach who will come and work with him. He'll have a fielding coach. He'll have a running coach.

Basically, the organization's whole focus is on helping players maximize their already built-in skill set, intelligence, and so on. That's what Jesse's life is like right now, and it's what his life will be like his entire playing career in baseball. That's a tremendous investment to make, but after all, the future sits with Jesse Winker.

Let's talk about somebody who's already walked through the minor leagues and hit the major league level: Johnny Cueto. He is a pitcher at the major league level and quite a good one at that. Johnny Cueto is going to have the same kind of support Jesse Winker has, but because Johnny Cueto is a pitcher, his responsibilities are different. So while Jesse is going to have to go out 130 times a year, Johnny will have to go out to the mound between 30 and 35 times a year. When he's not pitching, the other four days, he might limber up. He might throw. He's definitely going to get trained.

The organization is going to make sure Johnny eats right, works on his strength and conditioning, does his athletic training. The players will be fed before the game when they get to the ballpark and offered a robust food selection after every game. They'll have something for Johnny to do every single day, as well as studying the other teams, studying the batters, etc. (much like a surgeon studies all the diagnostic material before taking on a new case so they can do the best job possible by knowing their patient). That will be Johnny Cueto's life for as long as he plays major league baseball.

Now, let's talk about physicians. Dr. Pamela Hodul, who operated on my sister September 12, 2014, was in the operating room 13 and 1/2 hours. It was Friday, early evening, when she came out of surgery. It was a very difficult surgery, and Dr. Hodul actually cried. Both physically and emotionally, she was exhausted. She said she had told Susan she would do everything she could, and she felt she had.

But compare Dr. Hodul's support to the support provided to Jesse Winker and Johnny Cueto. What type of nutrition do you think she'll get? What type of conditioning training has she had to prepare her to handle this type of situation? What type of rub-down will she get from a trainer? Most likely what she'll get is a hard bagel and a cold cup of coffee before she goes home so she can grab a few hours of sleep before she has to do rounds the next day.

Imagine the stress physicians have when they lose patients. Cam Underhill was a "fire starter" at Baptist Easley Hospital in South Carolina. When she passed away, I was honored to be asked to go to Easley, SC, to do her eulogy. I saw her physician at the funeral, and he told me how terrible he felt when Cam had come to see him and he knew her cancer was metastasized. Another physician I heard talk said when he had to give a family such tragic news, all he could think about was that the patient was the same age as his wife and that his children were also the same age as this patient's children.

Losing patients is very hard and often very personal, and physicians carry this stress and pain with them. Now, think out of the box. What if, in medical school, a psychologist was assigned who could talk to them about failure, about stress, about grief, and about how to handle it all? What if a nutritionist was assigned to work with them? What if a strength and conditioning coach was provided, because physicians have unbelievable physical demands placed on them? What if they had a feedback loop like an athlete or an actor or anyone else who gets consistent feedback on their performance, what they do well and what they could do better? This makes perfect sense, doesn't it?

The big question that I've been getting as I travel the country to talk about this is, "Do you think physicians will really go for this approach to managing their health and wellness?" The answer is yes. Research has already indicated that they are open to the idea. In an article published in *Physician Executive Journal* titled "Physician Stress and Burnout: What Can We Do?", author Alan Rosenstein shares the results of a survey that tells us what physicians want. And what they want is ancillary support for administrative tasks, on-site exercise facilities, and wellness programs.[1]

Physicians are extremely dedicated hard workers and want to do what they need to do to make sure they can provide the best possible care for their patients. Physicians are amazing self-starters, and if offered a collegial, understanding environment, they thrive. Many will do their wellness endeavors on their own when pointed to a variety of sources; many, however, have voiced a desire for ongoing wellness activities. It is necessary to provide them to the best of our ability.

If physicians begin thinking about health and wellness when they're young, then it is easier to have their support for life. Start with medical students and residents, and they'll get used to it. Even if they don't see that nutritionist or the sports psychologist for a while, when they need them, they'll think, *Remember, the nutritionist told me this, that sports psychologist told me that,* and so on.

Some medical schools are already venturing into this territory. The Institute of Medicine, Education, and Spirituality at Ochsner (IMESO), initiated by the Ochsner Health System, is extending the definition of wellness to encompass a focus on students' inner lives. IMESO says its specialty is "to emphasize meaning and purpose in the life of each employee, which includes the integration of mind, body, and spirit in the workplace and the values that drive the organization."[2] It also reports that a course on reflective practice, which is taught by IMESO-trained physicians, was approved by the Ochsner Clinical School and the University of Queensland School of Medicine.

It's clear that our industry's education system is beginning to take physician wellness seriously and is willing to try new "out-of-the-box" approaches to help students create the foundation they need to avoid burnout.

Wellness programs have become a more common component and employee benefit in our workplace today with organizations requiring yearly wellness visits for every employee. However, this is not as common with physicians. In fact, it is not unusual for physicians to self-diagnose and to treat themselves.

With that in mind, a large hospital system in Texas implemented a requirement that all employees have a wellness check with their primary care physician each year. After a few years, they realized they were not requiring the same for employed physicians. So they are implementing a wellness check requirement for physicians as well. They actually found that a number of physicians did not have a primary care physician but were instead acting as their own physicians. The system feels these wellness checks for physicians is an important part of overall health and wellness for their physician staff and will be able to screen for issues such as burnout, anxiety, stress, and depression that might otherwise go undetected. They are even tying these wellness checks to their payroll and incentives.

I was at a health system in a small community that didn't have an athletic club or a YMCA available in their town. To help promote community health and wellness, the hospital built a fitness center attached to the hospital. It had a swimming pool, a weight room, an exercise room, a yoga room, and a full line of state-of-the-art cardio and strength training equipment. Although it was open to the community most of the time, they closed it off for three or four hours a day just for physicians to use.

Number one, physicians liked it not because they felt "elite" but because it functioned as sort of a safety net. They could talk freely with colleagues who understood the issues they were facing. Number two, they discovered they ended up having good conversations in there. It was a type of "talk therapy." Number three, they got in better shape and started feeling better, and they were appreciative that the hospital was providing this. So this is just one small example of what can happen when thinking out of the box regarding physician wellness.

I was speaking with a group of healthcare leaders and I brought up some of these wellness ideas for the physicians. One of the first questions I received was, "Quint, how can we afford a nutritionist? How can we afford to hire these kinds of people?" I said, "Think about it like this. What would happen if every physician could be more effective and more productive, and you could improve clinical quality, physician engagement, and access? How many new patients would you have to add to pay for this? How much cost would you really have to incur to pay for it?"

This is the kind of thinking I'm talking about when I say "out of the box." Wellness resources are not really expenses; they are investments that pay off many times over.

We're pretty lucky here in Pensacola. There is a flight team called the Blue Angels who are intensively trained. Well, our physicians are very much in this league; they are a professional championship team. If physicians are treated well and provided with resources they need to function at their highest level, it will more than pay for itself over and over again.

This is not only a financial matter, but a matter of serving the healthcare needs of the community. And it's a matter of making sure that not only our current physicians are kept engaged and aligned, but create an environment that will attract the next generation and the generation after that of the best and the brightest into the medical field to serve as physicians.

Physician Support Groups

A few things we're calling "out of the box" aren't really out of the box anymore.

In San Antonio, Texas, at Methodist Healthcare, Dr. George Ford has been studying this issue of burnout for years, and we were able to come together to share this passion. (You'll see on the cover that *Healing Physician Burnout* was written in collaboration with Dr. Ford.) Dr. Ford has been conducting seminars at the six campuses of the Methodist Hospital System. They have been very well attended and received by physicians, nurses, and the administration.

The first part of the three-fold focus has been to explain the epidemic of burnout and its negative impact upon healthcare delivery. The second focus has been to bring tools and tactics to clinicians for practical day-to-day application. The medical literature has expanded dramatically in the last two years regarding treatment modalities, and Dr. Ford has adapted his presentations to take into account these advances. He has also developed relationships with burnout experts nationally to share ideas. The third focus has been an effort to foster a healthcare environment receptive to honest and safe dialogue about burnout and its consequences. It is paramount to note that the administration has been very gracious in support of all of these endeavors.

Support groups have worked everywhere else and worked well. There are groups for substance abusers, people whose loved ones are suffering from Alzheimer's, people who have eating disorders, people whose children have autism, etc. If it's an issue people struggle with, there's probably a support group for it. So why shouldn't there be support groups for physicians and their (very real) struggles?

Sometimes finding out we're not alone can be a beautiful thing. I'm not saying that a 12-step program should be invented for physicians, but it might be a good idea to create a safe environment for them to come in and share what they're feeling, what's going on in their lives, and how they might handle the losses that they're feeling. And physicians do experience lots of losses—from the loss of their independence, to the loss of control over their work, to the loss of patients they cared deeply about.

Organizations that offer these types of services are going to win. Even physicians who don't take advantage of support groups are going to feel good that those are offered. You might say, "We have a big medical staff, but only a few physicians go to those things." Well, first of all, it costs almost nothing to set up a support group. And if you save one physician's life, you save the many patients they're responsible for. Isn't that what caring for the community is all about?

Professional Development Feedback Systems (Taking the Provider Feedback System^{SM} to the Next Level)

I was talking to a cardiovascular surgeon visiting Pensacola at a Pensacola Blue Wahoos baseball game. It happened by chance that Jeff Graupe, the director of player development for the Cincinnati Reds, was at the game. He had his laptop with him, and I asked if he would show this surgeon how they tracked the performance of their minor league players and what they do with that information. As the cardiovascular surgeon reviewed the data, he was just amazed. He saw how the baseball organization tracked every single player and their performance, and he saw the skill development plan for every single player.

Can this be duplicated for physicians? The fact is, physicians are very self-motivated individuals, so they do a great job keeping themselves up-to-date clinically. One of the most impressive things about physicians is that even when finances get tight, they don't cut training. Physicians have always kept a high standard for CME development because they understand how important it is to stay abreast of clinical changes for quality of patient care. Yet there are other areas besides clinical in which physicians benefit from development.

What if a best practice from minor league baseball was used and on a regular basis time was taken to create a professional development plan for physicians?

Sometimes when a physician graduates from medical school, they are seen as a "finished product." However, they are not. There seems to be an understood need for ongoing development in clinical advancement, so let's also focus on other needs. Today, physicians are expected to have much more knowledge of teamwork than ever before. An organization suddenly decides to implement Lean, and physicians need to be experts on patient flow. They need to have technology skills for the new electronic medical record. They're asked to use problem-solving skills in ways they never have before.

It would be really exciting if time was taken with physicians on a regular basis to create a professional development plan to track their progress and performance— much like other industries do for their elite performers. It doesn't make sense that development plans are created for almost everybody else in the healthcare system, but not for physicians. One can learn a lot from how other industries invest in, develop, and track their performers.

If a physician makes $200,000 a year with benefits, over a five-year period that comes to a million dollars. Let's compare these dollars to purchasing a piece of equipment. Certainly spending a million dollars on a piece of equipment is important and worth a lot of due diligence in the selection. However, this effort wouldn't stop there. A machine would not be bought and installed only to have the organization just move on. Instead, the organization would check up on it, maintain it, make sure it was being interacted with properly, maybe look at enhancements for it, and so forth.

The same should be true with physicians. Once physicians are part of the healthcare team, opportunities to help them continue to perform at a maximum level should be provided. This is done to enhance their professional life. Their personal life also benefits. When both areas are working well together, physicians are far less likely to burn out and far more likely to thrive.

Opportunities for Physician Collegiality

Peer relationships are important. Talking face-to-face with people who "get" us, who understand what our life is like, and who can commiserate with us, share ideas, and just plain bond is needed by us all. Physicians are no different. They need that sense of belonging that only regular, sustained, meaningful contact with their peers provides. Today, however, opportunities for physician collegiality are few and far between.

Imagine what a shock to the system this must be for physicians. Most were on some kind of "team" throughout their young lives. Maybe they played sports, or were on the debate team, or belonged to an academic society. Then, when they went to college and medical school, they continued to work closely with peers in groups or teams. During residency they also worked on very tight-knit teams. But when they joined a health system, suddenly, all that changed.

In their new role, physicians may work in teams with nurses and other healthcare professionals, but this does not yield the same conversations as talking with other physicians. Perhaps they even joined the health system specifically because they were recruited by another physician they liked or admired, but once hired they rarely if ever see that physician anymore. They can feel isolated and even lonely. And in the absence of collegial interaction, they may be more likely to burn out.

The loss of the time-honored physician lounge or if there is a lounge, loss of time to be in it, is a good symbol for what is happening. At one time physicians were in and out of the lounge often, discussing cases, chatting, having a cup of coffee, and so forth. Now, the pace of healthcare has sped up so much that the only thing that gets done in the physician lounge is work—if, that is, the lounge is even available.

Health systems must find a way to encourage and enable physician collegiality and camaraderie. Whether we reestablish physician lounges or establish physician "clubs" around books or other common interests, we need to do all we can to bring physicians together. Their well-being, and of course the well-being of the entire healthcare team and ultimately the patients, depends on it.

Many organizations are having success at creating this kind of environment. Advocate Good Samaritan Hospital in Downers Grove, Illinois, is a good example. In 2004, they launched a journey to performance excellence with a strategic intention to become the best place for physicians to practice, associates to work, and patients to receive care. Becoming the *best* place for physicians meant creating a culture of trust, collegiality, and collaboration. That culture began with a shift in how physicians were viewed—appreciating what they do, recognizing the challenges they face, and valuing the weighty responsibility they assume in caring for patients every day.

Secondly, they listened to the physicians' world and hearts to understand what was important to them—uncompromising quality, consistency of nursing expertise, efficiency of operations, economic success, exceptional experience for their patients, and inclusion in decisions and direction of the organization. Acting on what is important to physicians created a formula for breakthrough improvement and a powerful partnership. This effort resulted in some of the best risk-adjusted clinical outcomes in America and created a hospital where physicians not only want to practice but choose to bring their families for care.

Dave Fox, president of Advocate Good Samaritan, recently forwarded me this email, which does a beautiful job of showcasing how well their efforts have paid off:

Hello, Mr. Fox and Dr. Derus,

I would just like to compliment you both on your ongoing excellent work of nurturing and enfolding the medical staff here at Good Samaritan Hospital. I was privileged to attend a portion of the annual medical staff meeting last evening, to do a short presentation with our clinical informatics and IS team.

I see an awesome group of physicians gathering together as a "team," with both longevity (a lot) and newness to Good Sam. Physicians from many departments were represented, and it seems like they want to be a part of Good Samaritan's living organism in Downers Grove! I see them mingling and encouraging one another, mixing at different tables, and I see both of you extending yourselves to greet and enjoy their attendance also.

You work to make Good Sam a "home" for our excellent physicians to work, grow, serve, and be recognized for their investment in their own life and career and in the lives of the patients they touch every day, from their offices or here at Good Sam.

Thank you for making it obvious that you care for them as individuals, as much as for the work that they do here at Good Sam.

Keep up the good work. These are changing times, and this good journey will always need great people like you.

Mary Ziegler

Physician Liaison

Clinical Informatics

Good Samaritan Hospital

There will always be work to do toward creating great work environments for physicians, getting them aligned and engaged, and helping them alleviate and treat burnout—but when letters like this start coming in, we know that we are on the right path.

CHAPTER TWELVE:

PHYSICIAN, HEAL THYSELF: TACTICS FOR PHYSICIANS TO APPLY AT WORK AND HOME

W hile many of the tactics in this book are designed to be implemented by organizations, I want to speak directly about what you, the physician on the "front lines," can do to prevent, cope with, and reverse burnout in your own career.

Yes, your organization's culture has a significant impact on your energy, engagement, and mental health. But according to the *Emergency Medicine Journal*, a physician's individual coping style also has a significant impact on job performance, well-being, patient outcomes, and—yes—the likelihood of burnout.[1]

No matter what systems your organization may already have in place to mitigate the risk of physician burnout, you can and should take an active role in positively influencing your own mental, emotional, and physical health. The harder you work, the more important it is to properly manage yourself professionally and personally. And I know your workload is incredibly challenging and stressful. You owe it to yourself—not to mention your colleagues, staff, patients, and loved ones—to "heal yourself" as much as possible.

Let's take a look at three areas to focus on as you develop healthy coping mechanisms.

Tactics to Apply at Work

The following tactics can be applied at work to help stave off burnout.

Talk about what you're feeling and experiencing. A *New York Times* article by Pranay Sinha notes that "there is a strange machismo that pervades medicine." Not only are many physicians reluctant to share personal limitations and challenges; they often feel compelled to project physical, mental, and emotional capabilities beyond what they actually possess. As Sinha puts it, "We masquerade as strong and untroubled professionals even in our darkest and most self-doubting moments. How, then, are we supposed to identify colleagues in trouble— or admit that we may need help ourselves?"[2]

One of the first and most important steps is simple: Talk about it. Share your doubts, fears, and challenges with trusted colleagues. You will almost certainly hear two powerful words in response: "Me too." Knowing that you are not alone will bring you comfort and will also help you to forge a stronger connection with your peers. You may also find that older colleagues who have already been through these storms will act as mentors by sharing solutions and tactics.

Don't worry about seeming too vulnerable. Honesty and transparency, coupled with empathy and compassion, will benefit the medical community much more than pretending that everything is great. I encourage you to read the physician testimonies in Part 5 of this book to see that others have also struggled with burnout.

Speak up if you think you need help. If you notice that you are experiencing indicators of burnout, many of which are described in Chapter 7 of this book, go to a leader and let them know that you're struggling. Leaders may be able to help you identify the problem and determine how best to address it. As a former hospital executive, I can assure you that leaders are well aware of the pressures and risks that come with being on the front lines of healthcare, and know that it is in the best interests of the organization, patients, and physicians to address the causes and symptoms of burnout when they appear.

Also, don't hesitate to seek professional help outside of your hospital or organization—preferably before your burnout reaches crisis mode. A spiritual counselor, psychotherapist, or career coach can be a valuable resource in combating burnout and maintaining health.

Allow yourself to take regular vacations. With an ever-increasing workload, not to mention the responsibility you feel for your patients, this isn't always easy. I know of many physicians whose vacation time collects unused because they can't, or feel they shouldn't, leave.

But as much as possible, I encourage you to take vacations. If you were to ask your patients, I strongly suspect they would prefer to see an engaged, energized physician who is unavailable for short periods throughout the year, rather than a tired, stressed-out, unenthusiastic care provider who never takes a break.

If you still tend to think of vacation as a luxury or indulgence instead of a necessity, consider Medscape's 2015 Physician Lifestyle Report. It reveals that 36 percent of burned-out physicians take two weeks of vacation or less per year, and 5 percent have no vacation at all.[3]

Try to find a healthy work-life balance. While not always easy, this is very important in preventing burnout. No matter our professions, we all need time to decompress from work-related stress, to spend time with loved ones, and to engage in personal interests and responsibilities. If you don't take control of your time as much as you can, not only do you hurt your own health but you also neglect friends, family, and other commitments. This can cause you to become distracted and resentful when you are at work.

The good news is, taking steps to control your work schedule can have a positive impact on your job satisfaction and resilience. In one pilot study, physicians reported that knowing and setting limits, which included changing and restricting their practices, helped them achieve balance (and by extension, avoid burnout).[4] Do what you need to do to carve out time for yourself outside of work.

Take responsibility for your own training and development. This may help in two ways. One, you'll gain skills—whether they are administrative, technical, or pertaining to leadership—that make your day less stressful and more rewarding. Don't hesitate to approach leaders with ideas and requests to help you become more capable, efficient, and engaged. They will almost certainly welcome your input.

Second, a common indicator of burnout is a feeling of powerlessness over your environment. The very act of taking charge makes you feel more empowered and in control.

Seek a collaborative, engaged relationship with administrators. Sometimes a "we/they" relationship exists between physicians (and other frontline staff) and organizational leaders. When these two groups are disconnected, physicians can feel that they aren't appreciated, that their skills and abilities aren't being used to their full advantage, and that they are forced to spend their time on the "wrong" tasks.

That's why seeking a positive relationship with health system leaders is important. You will have an active voice in decisions and will be able to provide input in how things get done—which, in turn, may lessen the conditions that lead to burnout.

Give credit where it's due (especially with staff members). Treat staff and colleagues how you yourself would like to be treated. Dr. Starla Fitch writes, "…in this hurry-up world, we often don't thank people for helping out or stepping up. Studies show that people are willing to take a substantial cut in pay (up to $30K less, in some studies) to receive positive acknowledgment."[5]

As described in *Essentials for Great Patient Experiences* by Wendy Leebov, Dr. Randy Cook has experienced first-hand the power of positive acknowledgment. Leebov writes, "Dr. Cook praises his staff glowingly and appreciates very little turnover...He reinforces often that every staff member is important to building and sustaining relationships with patients and their families...He also feels very strongly that every person who enters their practice's doors should be treated with kindness, dignity, and respect, whether they are patients, family members, or colleagues. Consciously trying to model the behaviors expected of staff and complimenting people on them, Dr. Cook appreciates that his entire team shares and shows the practice's priority on patient-centered care and service."[6]

What does all of this have to do with burnout? It's simple: Staff turnover (not to mention their everyday attitudes) has a huge impact on physicians' stress levels and morale. When you put forth effort to create and maintain positive, appreciation-based relationships at work, you make it less likely that people will leave. Plus patient care improves, which also reduces physician stress and makes burnout less likely.

Think of patients as partners. Whether they don't understand their care plan or simply refuse to follow treatment recommendations, noncompliant patients are a big source of frustration for physicians. They can make physicians feel that they aren't making a difference. (This feeling is a classic indicator of burnout.) The solution is to engage patients as partners in their own care.

Leaders of the organizations coached by Studer Group® are asked to give patients a pen and piece of paper when they are in the waiting room. Patients are asked to write down any questions they may have, and also encouraged to take notes when speaking with their physicians. Even small tactics like this can give patients a stronger sense of ownership and help improve compliance, which reduces the likelihood of physician burnout.

Tactics to Apply in Your Personal Life

Chances are, few—if any—of these tactics will come as a complete surprise. Still, though, many physicians don't do them as often as they might. If you can get these basics right in your personal life, you'll find that the burnout needle moves in a positive direction.

Exercise regularly. Being in good physical shape helps you cope with stress and makes you feel better in general. Among other benefits, physical activity releases endorphins, boosts energy levels, improves your outlook, helps relax tense muscles and tissues, and improves the quality of your sleep. (I know you know this already and have probably shared this very information with your own patients. But for most of us, knowing and doing are two different things. It can sometimes help to be reminded!)

Remember that you don't have to train for a marathon or even have a gym membership to benefit from exercise. A 30-minute walk at least every other day can make a big difference in your quality of life. (If nothing else, that walk will get you out of the office, Emergency

Department, clinic, or wherever you practice for a much-needed break.) Of course, for physicians with hectic schedules, carving out 30 free minutes is easier said than done, but once you get the habit established, you'll find that the rewards are more than worth it.

Give back to others *off* the clock. As a physician you spend practically all of your working hours giving your time, talents, and expertise to others. You might assume that giving back to others when you are *off* the clock, too, will only hasten the onset of burnout. But this may not be the case. Medscape's 2015 Physician Lifestyle Report reveals that 37 percent of burned-out physicians never volunteer, while only 28 percent of non-burned-out physicians never volunteer.[7]

The nine-percentage-point difference between the two groups makes sense. As a recent *Forbes* article points out, volunteering has been found to improve health and happiness levels, lower depression rates, and even make practitioners feel as though they have more time.[8] The point? Finding an outside "cause" you care about—whether it is tutoring underprivileged children, rescuing animals, cleaning up local parks, or even engaging in medical mission work—can keep you connected to your passion and purpose at work, too.

Cultivate meaningful interests outside of work. If you read the physician testimonies in Part 5 of this book, you will see that a common thread is the recommendation to actively engage in fulfilling interests outside of work, whether that's playing a sport, painting, sailing, cooking, traveling, woodworking, playing a musical instrument, or something else.

Many physicians are in the habit of viewing hobbies as (at best) nice-to-have activities or (at worst) unnecessary wastes of time. This is a misconception. Hobbies are actually incredibly important for mental and emotional well-being. Engaging in a meaningful hobby or interest helps you take your focus off work when you're not on the clock. Sometimes you will even find yourself in a state of "flow" where you forget entirely about other stressors and worries.

Depending on their nature, hobbies might also improve your physical health, encourage a rich social life, and sharpen your mental processes—all of which stave off burnout. (The good news is, when you improve your work-life balance and take more vacation time as I have advised earlier in this chapter, you won't find it as difficult to carve out time for these healthy outlets.)

Find a healthy financial balance. One thing's for sure: Medical school tuition isn't getting any cheaper. There may not be a lot physicians can do to reduce the amount of student debt they carry. That's why it's especially important to avoid taking on too much debt in other arenas (like a huge mortgage) and to focus on creating a reasonable amount of savings. The impact of financial stress on one's mental and even physical health is well known.

"Burnout appears to have some association with physicians' view of their assets—or lack of them," writes Carol Peckham in Medscape's 2015 Physician Lifestyle

Report. "In the current report, 39 percent of burned-out physicians consider themselves to have minimal savings to unmanageable debt, compared with 28 percent of their less-stressed peers. Only 56 percent of burned-out physicians believe that they have adequate savings or more, compared with 66 percent of their less-stressed peers."[9]

Focus on nurturing, not managing, your relationships. At work, you expect your team to be high performers who act with initiative and who can be trusted to carry out their responsibilities to the very highest standards. When this isn't the case, there are consequences. After all, the well-being of your patients—sometimes, their very lives—depends on your staff's performance.

Often, physicians may unconsciously bring these high expectations home and find it stressful when their spouses, children, friends, and neighbors don't live up to them. Now, I believe that what you permit, you promote, and would never encourage you to overlook or condone bad behavior. However, I *do* encourage you to take a fresh look at your relationships outside of work. Try to nurture and grow the relationships that are most important to you.

Mental Resources to Develop

Whether you are at work or at home, the more control you have over your thoughts and mindset, the less likely you will be to succumb to burnout.

Be aware of the benefits of stress. The word "stress" is so often used in a negative way that it is easy to forget its positive aspects. For instance, as a physician, you are aware that the human body is actually strengthened when progressive stress is applied to muscles and the cardiovascular system. For most of us, this is exactly our goal when we go into the gym to exercise. However, when building strength, the key to success is applying stress in small incremental doses, as excessive stress will break down muscle.

The same thing is true of the stress you encounter in your work as a physician. In manageable amounts, challenges and pressure can help build your resilience, knowledge, and stamina. You may find it helpful to remind yourself of this truth when the going gets tough. (Yet the line between helpful and harmful stress *does* exist, and it differs for each person. Don't keep pushing yourself if you are exhibiting the indicators of burnout described in Chapter 7 of this book.)

Maintain emotional self-awareness. Burnout does not happen overnight; it builds over a long period of time. However, many of its indicators and symptoms can sneak up on physicians. Especially since it is so easy to become swept up in the frantic pace of providing care these days, physicians should focus on maintaining self-awareness at all times.

At regular intervals—even if it's pausing for only half a minute between patient appointments—stop, close your eyes, and assess how you're feeling. If you are frustrated, upset, or anxious, try to determine the cause.

Just knowing *why* you are feeling a certain way can help you put your emotions into perspective so that they don't cause you continued stress. This tactic can also help you to maintain more productive, fulfilling relationships with patients and colleagues because it will prevent you from venting any negativity you feel on people who aren't the cause.

Practice mindfulness techniques. Medicine is an inherently demanding occupation, and it isn't always possible to reduce or eliminate the stressors physicians encounter. However, you *can* take steps to manage the nature and duration of your response to stress. According to Dr. George Ford, one of the most effective ways to manage your thoughts, actions, and reactions is developing mindfulness. Defined as "paying attention in a particular way, on purpose, in the present moment, and nonjudgmentally,"[10] mindfulness can help physicians create a sense of objectivity and acceptance in the face of life's unavoidable frustrations.

In the seminars he conducts to explore and address the issue of burnout, Dr. Ford teaches mindfulness techniques adapted from the Rochester Medical School model by Mick Krasner and Ron Epstein. On your own, you can use cognitive-behavioral training, meditation, massage, breathing exercises, and more to increase your mindfulness, and thus your ability to manage your thoughts, actions, and reactions.

Also, more and more physicians are advising patients to turn to yoga, tai chi, qigong, and other mind-body therapies to relieve stress and promote mindful wellness.

There's a reason that so many physicians are turning to methods once considered "alternative": They work.

All of the tactics I have shared in this chapter are effective ways for physicians to prevent, combat, and reverse burnout. To start, I encourage you to choose a few strategies that appeal most to you or that address a problem you have been experiencing. Focus on really incorporating those strategies into your life and pay attention to how your attitude and outlook change.

To close this chapter that aims to help you "heal thyself," I would like to leave you with one more well-known medical saying: "An ounce of prevention is worth a pound of cure." You know that this proverb is full of wisdom, and you adhere to its implications in your practice. You would never advise a patient to wait until his joint pain became debilitating before prescribing medication and physical therapy. You would never tell someone with cardiovascular disease risk factors that there is no need to make lifestyle changes unless she experienced a heart attack.

So please, show yourself the same courtesy and be proactive about safeguarding your well-being. Don't tell yourself that you can "tough it out" or that "this too shall pass." It's much better to address burnout *before* it happens.

PART FIVE:

PROFILES IN PASSION AND PURPOSE: HOW PHYSICIANS PREVENT, COPE WITH, AND HEAL FROM BURNOUT

DR. GEORGE FORD: MY BURNOUT STORY

D *r. George A. Ford, III, is in his 35th year of private practice in internal medicine at iMED Healthcare Associates in San Antonio, Texas. He is an adjunct professor of internal medicine at the University of Texas Health Science Center at San Antonio, in which capacity he has served as clinical preceptor for medical students and residents for over 25 years. He is very involved in the Bioethics Committee of the Methodist Healthcare System in a consulting and teaching capacity. He is on the Medical Executive Committee at Methodist Stone Oak Hospital and is chairman of the Physician Resource Committee. It is in this role that he serves as physician advocate, deals with behavioral issues, and utilizes his experience with burnout.*

I started the private practice of internal medicine 35 years ago, with the typical idealism of a young physician. I had the "Peace Corps mindset" of wanting to make the world a better place. I joined an excellent group in San Antonio and worked hard to build a good practice. Initially, the energy required to keep everything moving forward was fueled by enthusiasm and most importantly *The Call.*

About 10 years into practice, I found myself saying to the medical students and residents I mentored that I had developed a "love-hate" relationship to medicine. At one level, I could hardly believe that I was capable of saying such a thing, let alone believing it! It just seemed that it required more and more energy to keep all those plates spinning. My existential state was analogous to walking into the surf: initially easy and refreshing, but then the deeper I went, I found myself buffeted not only by the visible waves on the surface, but even more by the invisible undertow. Equanimity began to be replaced by **exhaustion**, **cynicism**, and a decaying **sense of purpose**.

For a two-year period, I would use the weekend to gear up for the week, then be depleted by the end of the week. I felt like a grape on Mondays, and by Fridays my vitality was drained and I felt like a raisin. For a two-year period I seriously contemplated leaving medicine. But to what?

The crucible of this two-year period culminated in a deeply spiritual "dark night of the soul" and then blossomed into my Christian faith. This rebirth set me on my way to see everything through different eyes. Appropriate perspective replaced a need to "fix things"; insoluble existential crises with my patients could be seen as opportunities for enrichment of the doctor-patient relationship.

The crucible of crisis is never enjoyed when it is operant, but it would not serve its purpose were that the case. Life's challenges are designed to challenge one's individual resources and problem-solving skills. They serve to beckon one to a larger agenda and purpose. *The Call* serves as the clarion to spur one on past the point of discomfort at which one might otherwise quit.

Emotional exhaustion was now replaced with a sense of curiosity and anticipation for what each visit might bring. I became open to the possibility of exciting trails to follow.

Cynicism (***depersonalization***) was also quickly dispatched as new bridges of communication were opened with my patients and their families. The narratives into which their lives were embedded became distinctive and important to me.

As for my ***sense of purpose***, it had been rekindled. I was now empowered, having survived the crucible of life experience, to realize the full implication of my *Call*. I found that I particularly enjoyed counseling my patients, especially those physicians and nurses who came in for examination. They would never announce a diagnosis of burnout, but would present with the characteristic symptoms. As I looked into their eyes, the "windows of the soul," I saw little evidence of the spark of life. However, when I would direct them back to their youthful passion, long since forgotten, I was able to relight the pilot light. That would allow the passion to begin to flow again.

I truly enjoyed counseling my patients and colleagues who manifested burnout. At one point about 10 years ago, I heard about a colleague who had been so despairing that he had attempted suicide. To this I announced to my ethics colleagues a desire to do something formal for a wider audience of colleagues.

It was at this juncture when I inquired among a group of colleagues at a national ethics conference at Georgetown University, indeed not even having been acquainted with the word "burnout"(!), that Providence again intervened. Through gracious colleagues, I was introduced to several experts in the field of burnout in the U.S. and Canada. I began devouring every article and book that I could find. I began leading seminars on burnout diagnosis and treatment to my colleagues in San Antonio. The leaders of the Methodist Hospital System here in San Antonio were enthusiastic supporters.

It was rewarding to find that the literature of burnout treatment endorsed many of the things that I was already doing during the previous 15 years. I was amazed to find that Dr. Christina Maslach's tripartite definition of burnout (emotional exhaustion, depersonalization, and loss of sense of purpose) described perfectly my prior existential crisis. I was able to speak with her about her journey, and she connected me with her partner, Dr. Michael Leiter, who came to San Antonio and worked with our group for a six-month period.

I approached Mr. Studer about five years ago at a national Studer Group® conference in Dallas. I told him that I had not read anything about burnout in his books. An instant look of recognition flashed from his eyes, as if something burning deep within his soul was now given expression. He told me to get together with him, that burnout might just be the next big item to report.

We have spoken numerous times and dialogued about burnout, gathering information and watching the growth of the literature on burnout.

The literature has literally exploded in the last two years, and we both felt that the time was perfect, as burnout has even received exposure in the literature and media (such as the *New York Times*).

The rest, as they say, is history. And you have in your hands this book that truly represents a "labor of love" for both Mr. Studer and myself. He has been magnanimous in extending to me this opportunity to work with him as a colleague.

Much more is to be written, but a pathway toward healing is now clearly in front of us.

George A. Ford, III, MD, FACP

Dr. Samuel Harris: The Importance of Putting Stress in Perspective

D r. *Samuel T. Harris graduated from St. George's University School of Medicine. He works in Knoxville, TN, and specializes in internal medicine. Dr. Harris is affiliated with Team Health and works at Roane Medical Center.*

Sometimes when life is tough it can help to consider the plight of those who have it much worse than you do. A difficult childhood in an impoverished, war-torn Liberia has given Dr. Samuel Harris a sense of perspective regarding the stresses of practicing medicine in 21st century America.

Dr. Harris saw close friends and family suffer from the lack of good medical care available in his homeland. Because of these experiences, he vowed to become a physician so he would never be powerless in that way again. Now, while there are certainly times he feels overwhelmed and underappreciated (like all physicians), he recalls the trials that inspired him to choose this profession in the first place.

"I do get burned out, but I always go back to where I came from," he says. "I think about the days when we had no food to eat. We had to set traps to catch animals to feed ourselves. We had no hospitals, no clinics. I say to myself, 'This is nothing in comparison. I can take this.' I just take it one day at a time."

Dr. Harris maintains his perspective and passion for patient care by regularly returning to Liberia. There, he visits the villages and sets up clinics for those without access to medical care. For him, it's a way to remember the big picture behind the everyday difficulties of being a doctor.

"It reminds me not to forget where I was raised," he explains. "Not to forget the pains I've been through, the people and circumstances I grew up with. I've been blessed to have come so far. I go back to give back."

These visits remind him never to take the life he has now—life itself, for that matter—for granted.

"Every time I go back, I'm reminded over and over again how brittle life is," he says. "In a snap, just like that, it's gone."

Because of his experiences and passion for helping people, Dr. Harris takes special care to make patients feel at ease. By taking the time to talk with and learn about them, he has a chance to relax during demanding days at the hospital and reconnect with the human element that first drew him to medicine.

"One complaint I hear a lot from patients is that the doctor doesn't give them much time," he says. "He's got one foot in the door, one out the door. When you sit down, you give the person the impression that you are there for them. No matter how busy I am, that's my time to relax a bit. I sit down and say, 'Let's talk.' People connect with you more when they feel like you're genuinely interested in knowing what's going on with them and you really want to help."

Just like anyone else, Dr. Harris has days when he feels burdened by his work and all the sadness and pain that come with not being able to make every patient well. Yet if he ever questions that the medical field is where he belongs, he remembers the struggles he saw and experienced in Liberia.

"It affects me every single day in how I relate to people," he affirms. "I've seen both ends. I've lived where you have nothing, no healthcare, zero, and I have seen where you have everything and how you use or misuse it.

"I have rough days, too, but I try to just smile and laugh," he concludes. "Every now and then I'll frown and I'll come home and pray about it. For me, being a doctor is a duty. I have to do this because it's what I'm called to do."

Dr. Hogai G. Nassery: Too Much Stress Can Be Life-Threatening (Even When It's Fueled by Caring)

D*r. Hogai G. Nassery graduated from the Medical College of Georgia School of Medicine in 1994. She works in Atlanta, GA, and specializes in family medicine. Dr. Nassery works in the Grady Health System.*

Often, the people who care the most deeply are also the ones who are most vulnerable to the ravages of burnout. Dr. Hogai G. Nassery is a good example. Beginning with the work she did in an Afghan refugee camp at the age of 18, she has always been fiercely dedicated to effecting social change. That's why she spent more than a decade practicing medicine in underserved communities of Atlanta—a role that made each day incredibly rewarding.

Eventually, though, Dr. Nassery was asked to take on the role of Chief of Community Medicine—and that's when the stress began to take its toll on her health.

"I was a little torn about that decision because I had two small children," she recalls. "But the way I was raised, it wasn't easy for me to say no to an opportunity like that. To think that I could have more of an impact on people's lives—I felt I had to accept."

Before long, Dr. Nassery was overwhelmed with responsibilities. In addition to seeing patients, her administrative role had her teaching residents, negotiating contracts, hiring and training new physicians, covering clinics, writing up new policies and job descriptions, and more. Meanwhile, she was on the boards of two non-profit organizations.

"I was also so worried about serving my patients well," she says. "If it was hard for someone to get an appointment, I would feel so guilty, so angry. It seemed like letting down the community. I was personalizing everything to a degree that wasn't healthy."

During all this, she struggled to balance her personal life as well, taking care of her two young boys and a father with Parkinson's. She was devastated when he passed away, but continued to push herself out of an obligation to her patients, practice, and family.

"I remember covering in the clinic one particular afternoon and thinking to myself, *I cannot keep up this pace*," she recalls. "My administrative duties were becoming overwhelming. I knew I was in trouble, that I was overdoing it, but I just kept going."

One Friday, after giving a lecture and rushing to attend her older son's birthday party, she went to bed with abdominal pain. By the following Tuesday, she was unable to function. Her husband rushed her to the emergency room in shock, delirious and short of breath. She later found out that she had toxic shock syndrome, resulting in renal, respiratory, and heart failure, and GI bleeding. She spent three weeks in the hospital, hooked up to a ventilator for much of it, and says that it took six months to be able to function normally again.

"During this time of recovery, I had a lot of time to think," she says. "I realized I had been burning the candle at both ends. I was emotionally stressed because of my father's passing and was grieving deeply. I had no work-life balance. I was burned out.

"Thankfully, I had a tremendous amount of support from my colleagues," she comments. "While I was unconscious, they were at the hospital talking with my husband and doctors every day. They were just amazing. My infectious disease doctor said, 'Do you know everybody in Atlanta?' because all these doctors had been calling her from Grady and Emory, which was so heartwarming."

Looking back, Dr. Nassery realizes that she needed a wake-up call. Being responsible for patients' health is a formidable source of stress for any healthcare professional, and if internalized too deeply, it can have serious mental, emotional, and physical consequences.

"I think that had to happen at that point for me to stop and really reflect back on what I was doing," she says. "In some ways, it was really a blessing that it happened. I reevaluated and made some major changes in my life. I resigned from the boards I was on and became more mindful of my priorities—especially my husband and kids.

"Now, I have this inner sense of when I'm done at the end of the day that I didn't have back then," she concludes. "I remind myself that all I can do is what I can do. And if I'm struggling, I need to ask for help from my family, neighbors, or colleagues. It never serves anyone well to push themselves the way I used to."

DR. ALAN SHELTON: SPIRITUALITY, GRATITUDE, AND BALANCE CAN HELP HEAL BURNOUT

D*r. Alan Shelton is the clinical director at the Puyallup Tribal Health Authority in Tacoma, Washington, where he has worked as a family practitioner for over 30 years, serving the Native American Puyallup tribe. He also serves on the faculty at the Tacoma Family Medicine residency program at MultiCare Hospital in Tacoma, Washington.*

Growing up abroad as the son of a missionary family, Dr. Alan Shelton felt called to make a difference by practicing medicine from an early age. So it's not surprising that Dr. Shelton's career path led him to Tacoma, Washington, where he has worked with the Native American Puyallup tribe for over 30 years.

"When I arrived, the Puyallup tribe was very impoverished," Dr. Shelton recalls. "My ideals and energy carried me through the challenges of the first years, but over time, little by little, I felt myself changing. Twenty years in I had become the clinic's medical director, but I had trouble finding the motivation to get up and go to work. I felt hollow, cynical, and useless, and was plagued by a sense that nothing was good anymore."

Like many physicians, Dr. Shelton realized that he had crossed the line into burnout when he began to notice his own negative feelings toward many of his patients, who often came to him angry, bitter, and demanding because they were in pain.

"Most people think burnout is exhaustion—and it is—but it is much more than physical tiredness," he says. "Physicians who are burned out are mentally and emotionally exhausted, and no longer have the inner resources to deal effectively with difficulty, stress, and problems."

For Dr. Shelton, a turning point came when his staff asked him to meet with the Puyallup tribal shaman. Though he was initially reluctant, Dr. Shelton came away from the meeting having gained a transformative insight.

He says: "If you're physically healthy, the word to describe you is 'fit.' If you're emotionally healthy, it's 'adjusted.' And I learned that in the Native American community, the word to describe someone who has a healthy spirituality is 'connected.' This isn't about religion in the traditional sense, but about being in tune with some sense of the divine, with the world around you, and with other people. And it doesn't just happen automatically."

From that point on, Dr. Shelton concentrated on renewing his spirit and reconnecting to the community he longed to help. He found the power of mindful gratitude to be particularly healing.

"I realized that if I looked at the frustrating parts of my job in a different way, I could find some way to be thankful," he says. "At first I was thankful that things *could* have been a whole lot worse but weren't. Then, as my gratitude evolved and became a habit, I was thankful for situations that gave me the opportunity to learn, grow, and become more compassionate. Instead of allowing myself to become consumed by my patients' setbacks and difficulties, I began to focus on how wonderful it was to see them find a way, little by little, back to recovery and health."

Ultimately, the lesson Dr. Shelton has learned is that a life out of balance leads to burnout. He feels fortunate that in his own life, burnout became a helpful catalyst, a vehicle of revitalization and renewal. This, along with his deep respect for the Native American spiritual tradition, inspires him to share with other physicians the essential roles spirituality and connectedness play in achieving true satisfaction and fulfillment at work. In addition to conducting workshops, he has written *Transforming Burnout: A Simple Guide to Self-Renewal*, a book that teaches readers to find a healthy balance in body, mind, and spirit.

"It's so important for all physicians to realize that well-being is not dependent on situations, relationships, or any outer circumstance," Dr. Shelton notes. "It is directly related to the quality of your inner life. While spirituality and balance look different for everyone, it's crucial to address the causes and conditions that are disrupting them and to find a coping mechanism that reconnects you with passion, enthusiasm, and joy."

DR. DOUGLAS SMITH: TO AVOID ACCRUING AN "EMPATHY DEBT," PHYSICIANS MUST RECHARGE

D*r. Douglas Smith is the Executive Vice President of EmCare's Alliance Group. He has over 15 years of clinical leadership experience in medical staff development, emergency medicine, and healthcare informatics. At EmCare he is responsible for the management of multiple hospitals in the mid-Atlantic and northeast United States, with emergency medicine, hospitalist, psychiatric, and rehabilitation specialties. Dr. Smith also serves as an emergency physician in the U.S. Army Reserve and currently holds the rank of lieutenant colonel.*

Before accepting his position at EmCare, Dr. Smith worked full-time in clinical emergency medicine and describes those years as being full of rewarding moments. However, he also acknowledges that due to the frantic pace of the Emergency Department, he wasn't able to deeply connect with patients as often as he would have liked. Overall, his days were grueling and exhausting. In fact, even outside of work he found he lived (and still does, to some extent) in a state of hyper-alertness that is by itself inherently stressful.

"Emergency physicians live in a unique world," he says. "We are constantly preparing for what *could* go wrong. As I ride down the road with my wife in the car, I envision the school bus in front of me turning over and catching fire. I think about a deer coming through the windshield. It's just a constant state of preparation: What would I do? How would I respond?"

Dr. Smith says being perpetually "at the ready" prepares ED physicians to handle their emotions when such situations actually happen.

"Add to this the cases emergency physicians encounter on a daily basis, and you have a recipe for constant stress," he says. "Of course, each sick toddler, car crash victim, or patient death takes a toll, but you don't have time to process those emotions. Things move so quickly that you just have to bottle up what you feel, move to the next room, and deal with another situation."

Dr. Smith says that years of being unable to fully feel and express pain caused him to become frustrated and angry with patients and colleagues. Ultimately, the doctor he saw when he looked in the mirror was not who he wanted to be. That's when he realized he was burning out.

He now refers to what he felt and experienced as an "empathy debt." Over time, he says, physicians build an inner dam that allows them to hold back the stress, pain, and emotion caused by their careers. But eventually, the dam will break, and the debt *will* be paid.

"My own empathy debt was called in when my wife, Jennifer, was diagnosed with colon cancer," he recalls. "This crisis triggered the release of all of the emotions I'd built up. I was an absolute wreck. I cried in the car, I cried with the radio, I cried at her bedside. I cried and cried for days until years' worth of emotions were spent."

The point is, stress never just dissipates; it always finds its way out. In fact, says Dr. Smith, physicians see undealt-with stress aggravating their patients' chronic abdominal pain, migraines, Crohn's disease, and other conditions all the time.

"It's so important for physicians to have down time, to find an outlet that lets them manage their emotions and recharge," he says. "For me, it's sailing. For others, it might be reading, singing, prayer, running, playing golf, swimming, or traveling.

"And it's absolutely not just about recharging mentally so that you can think critically," he adds. "It's also recharging empathetically. It's about renewing your ability to care about what you're doing and whom you're doing it for in each situation."

Dr. Rodney O. Tucker: Meaning and Powerful Patient Connections Keep Physicians Recharged

D*r. Rodney O. Tucker has practiced medicine for over 25 years, working in private practice and palliative care. He currently serves as director for the Center for Palliative and Supportive Care at the University of Alabama at Birmingham (UAB) Medical Center and as the Chief Experience Officer for UAB Medicine.*

Burnout is a possibility for everyone who chooses the demanding, stressful medical profession. Yet physicians who avoid burnout, or at least bounce back from it when it occurs, often have a strong sense that they do meaningful work, coupled with powerful patient connections. Both have helped Dr. Rodney O. Tucker maintain his mental and emotional well-being over the years.

"Here's what inspired me to practice medicine," says Dr. Tucker. "You enter people's lives in ways that really only loved ones, spouses, children, and probably clergy and spiritual advisors are given the opportunity to do."

He says that through all the phases of his career, he has been able to draw new energy and purpose from the strong relationships he builds with his patients. He credits each of them with helping him to stay engaged in and passionate about his work as a physician.

Dr. Tucker initially discovered the power of the patient-physician relationship as a first-year medical student.

"At that time my grandfather was 96 years old, in a nursing home, and suffering from chronic pain," he recalls. "When I visited, he would tell the nurses that his grandson was a doctor (even though I wasn't yet), and would insist that I give him his shots (even though I had told him I wasn't yet qualified).

"Of course, when he turned over and looked the other way, the nurse would say, 'Okay, Rodney is giving you the shot,' while administering it herself. But my grandfather swore those shots worked better because I 'gave' them to him."

To his grandfather, that's what medicine was about: giving shots. In his mind, that's what doctors did. (In fact, says Dr. Tucker, "If I ever write a book, that will be the title: *Giving Shots*.")

"The point is, the fact that I was this man's grandson enhanced his perception of the quality of his care," he continues. "That experience is one reason why I chose the field of palliative care. It's also why I have always tried to make my relationships with patients not just about providing medical care, but about getting to know them personally and forming a bond of trust."

Not only does forging a stronger connection with patients enhance their care; it also carries deep rewards for physicians. Dr. Tucker recalls a recent patient whose routine care grew into a long and lasting friendship.

"This graceful, bright, poised woman came to me in her 70s for pain management, and unfortunately, early dementia crept in soon after," he says. "Her family asked me to be the 'quarterback' of her care to make her last years as comfortable and stress-free as possible."

Over the next seven years, Dr. Tucker grew to know his patient and her family well. He carries her story with him because he realized that the love her family had for her was more powerful than any medicine he could give. He recalls the positivity that filled the room when her grandchildren would hug her and when her husband would wink at her and talk about "his girl."

"As physicians, we all encounter situations like this—situations that have the power to inspire us and to connect us in meaningful ways with our patients," he comments. "If we look beyond the injury or condition or illness and see the person, we will be able to plug back into what makes this profession so meaningful."

CONCLUSION

I 've been so fortunate to work in healthcare. Over the past several decades, I've learned a lot about human beings in general and about healthcare professionals in particular, and one of the things I've learned is this: When people believe strongly in something and are fully invested in it, they can do amazing things.

That's why I am so certain that engagement and alignment are the keys to solving the physician burnout epidemic. Why? Because when physicians really buy into and get excited about an organization's mission, they will put the full force of their passion, intelligence, and caring behind that mission. When that happens, miracles can occur.

Burnout is really just a symptom of many big, complex issues—the massive changes happening in healthcare, challenges in how we train physicians, challenges in how we help them transition to new employment structures, and so forth. Healthcare has so many moving parts, all of which impact other parts, that solving all the challenges we face is going to be incredibly complicated.

We simply can't control what's happening in the external healthcare environment. We can't fix everything that needs fixing. But we can change what we *can* change in terms of how we lead and how our organizations operate. And we *can* reconnect physicians to the passion and purpose that lie at the heart of why they chose their profession in the first place. If we can do those two things, we can get some real momentum going.

That's another lesson I've learned from my work in healthcare. I've seen it over and over again: Once things get moving, they keep moving. They pick up steam. The results keep multiplying and escalating. That's the idea behind the Healthcare Flywheel® that I talk about to organizations coached by Studer Group® and that I've put on the covers of several books we've published. And once a flywheel gets started, it's very hard to stop.

At the hub of the Healthcare Flywheel is this phrase: "purpose, worthwhile work, and making a difference." The reason we placed it at the center is because it's what really is what drives all healthcare professionals, physicians included. Yet sometimes we all forget how passionate we felt when we started in this field and that is also true of physicians.

When I was researching this book I read a *Wall Street Journal* article by Sandeep Jauhar (himself a physician) titled "Why Doctors Are Sick of Their Profession." He said in it that the profession of medicine is in a midlife crisis and struggling with a sense of lost status. Where doctors were once "pillars of the community," now "the job has become only that—a job."

That statement really hit me. I thought how tragic it is that so many physicians feel this way. Now, I believe that *all* jobs, done well and in the right spirit, are worthwhile and noble. All jobs serve a purpose. But what higher purpose can there be than healing people and saving lives? It's hard to think of a line of work that should be richer, more rewarding, and more meaningful.

Also, no matter what a job is, when a worker is fully engaged in it, outcomes are better. Products and services are of higher quality. Customers are more satisfied. Companies are financially healthier. And of course the process of making those products and providing those services goes more smoothly. It just goes better for everyone involved.

Physicians need and deserve to feel great about what they do. In fact, we should all feel great about working in healthcare, but none of us can feel this way if physicians can't. (It reminds me of how if one part of the body is sick or not working right, the entire person feels bad.) We're all in this together and we all need to be happy and healthy. We all need to be aligned and engaged and working toward the same goals, the same mission.

The good news is there is a lot we can do inside our health systems to get physicians engaged and aligned. We can create great places for physicians to work, and this is the heart and soul of great healthcare. When we can meet the four physician drivers—if you'll recall, they are *quality, efficiency, input,* and *appreciation*—we are setting physicians up to be able to achieve the sense of purpose, worthwhile work, and making a difference that they need to thrive.

A great working environment and a great mindset is an unbeatable combination in a physician. It's also the winning formula for superior patient care and long-term organizational health.

When physicians thrive, we all thrive—healthcare organizations, team members, and, of course, patients and families. Let's work together to make it happen.

Quint

A SPECIAL THANK-YOU
TO GEORGE FORD, MD

Writing a book is always a collaborative effort. There are so many people behind the scenes who contribute in various ways to the finished work. In this case, I'd like to honor an individual who went "above and beyond" in assisting with *Healing Physician Burnout*.

Dr. George Ford has been an advocate for helping prevent and treat physician burnout for a long time. He was researching and writing about the subject years ago, long before it became such a hot topic. He truly is a thought leader in this area, and his passion on the subject is a big inspiration to me.

In fact, while physician burnout has been on my mind for many years, it was Dr. Ford who really helped me move from "thinking about" to "doing." After a particular situation occurred, I realized I need to do more in this area. It was about that same time that Dr. Ford called me.

Dr. Ford specializes in internal medicine at Methodist Healthcare in San Antonio, TX, an organization that Studer Group has been working with for some time. When he called me, he shared that he felt with the Studer Group reach, we were in a good position to shine more light on the subject of physician burnout. He also felt that many of our tools and techniques were useful in creating a better work environment for physicians.

This led to Dr. Ford and me filming a webinar on the subject of physician burnout as well as collaborating on a white paper titled "Physician Burnout: Preparing for a Perfect Storm," which was published by Studer Group in 2012. Also, through the years, Dr. Ford has provided many articles containing research on physician burnout.

Dr. Ford, along with Jaime Wesolowski, president and chief executive officer of the Methodist Healthcare System in San Antonio, will be in the forefront of making physician lives better.

Dr. Ford was incredibly valuable in helping research many of the issues covered in these pages and in connecting the dots in unusual and thought-provoking ways. He has a deep understanding of the implications of physician burnout and the urgency with which our industry needs to act, and his perspective has truly taken the content to the next level.

Thank you, Dr. Ford, for your dedication, enriching insights, and generous spirit. Your fingerprints can be found throughout this book.

In gratitude,

Quint

ACKNOWLEDGMENTS

T his book would not exist without the passion, focus, and hard work of those listed below.

Thank you to the physicians dedicated to their profession, the patients in their care, and the organizations committed to creating a great environment for physicians and all staff.

Margaret Stanzell, Dottie DeHart, and Bekki Kennedy have been a part of each of my books. Seven books together and the adventure continues...

To Margaret: Thank you for being the "pitching coach, hitting coach, and running coach" all rolled into one. Your spot-on attention to detail and impressive co-ordination of several drafts, edits, interviews, and much more was the unwavering force that made this book possible. You will always have "major league" standing with me.

To Dottie: This book would not have come to be without our partnership on making sure each phrase hits the right tone. Of course, thank you also to the DeHart & Company team for the countless hours they have put into making this book happen.

To Bekki: Every book we work on together is an adventure. Your insight and direction make each one an impactful resource for healthcare professionals everywhere.

To Jamie Stewart: Thank you for ensuring that all of the details happened to make this book a reality in the hands of those who will gain the greatest impact from it.

To Annalise Davis: Thank you for providing assistance at key times to keep this important content in front of me and moving forward.

To George Ford, MD: Thank you for the decades of dedication to the topic of physician burnout.

Thanks also to the difference-makers at Studer Group who continue to ignite my flame.

And, finally, thanks to all the Fire Starters who serve with such purpose, do worthwhile work, and make a difference.

REFERENCES

Part One Intro:

1. Jauhar, S., "Why Doctors Are Sick of Their Profession," *The Wall Street Journal* August 29, 2014.

2. Peckham, C., "Physician Burnout: It Just Keeps Getting Worse," *Medscape Physician Lifestyle Report* January 26, 2015.

3. Wicks, R. J., Overcoming Secondary Stress in Medical and Nursing Practice (Oxford University Press, 2006) 18.

4. "Physician Misery Index Survey," *Geneia*, March 5, 2015, http://www.geneia.com/news-and-events/geneia-survey/

5. Friedberg, M. et al., "Factors Affecting Physician Professional Satisfaction and Their Implications for Patient Care, Health Systems, and Health Policy," *Rand Corporation* 2013.

Chapter 1:

1. "National Health Expenditure Accounts," *Centers for Medicare & Medicaid Services*, last accessed June 30, 2015, http://www.cms.gov/Research-Statistics-Data-and-Systems/Statistics-Trends-and-Reports/NationalHealthExpendData/nationalHealthAccountsHistorical.html

2. Shanafelt, TD. et al., "Satisfaction with Work-Life Balance and the Career and Retirement Plans of U.S. Oncologists," *Journal of Clinical Oncology*, 2014, 32 (11): 1127-35. doi: 10.1200/JCO.2013.53.4560. Epub 2014 Mar 10.

3. Miller, P. et al., *In Their Own Words* (New York: Morgan-James, 2010) 15.

4. Barr, P., "The Boomer Challenge," *Hospitals & Health Networks*, January 14, 2014.

5. Mechanic, D., "Physician Discontent: Challenges and Opportunities," *JAMA*, August 20, 2003; 290 (7): 941-6.

Chapter 2:

1. "2014 Survey of American Physicians: Practice Patterns and Perspectives," *The Physicians Foundation by Merritt Hawkins*, September 2014. http://www.physiciansfoundation.org/uploads/default/2014_Physicians_Foundation_Biennial_Physician_Survey_Report.pdf.

2. Shanafelt, TD. et al., "Burnout and Satisfaction with Work-Life Balance Among US Physicians Relative to the General US Population," *Archives of Internal Medicine*, 2012, 172 (18): 1377-85.

3. "Survey Finds Rising 'Misery Index' Among Doctors," *NH Business Review*, April 3, 2015. http://www.nhbr.com/April-3-2015/Survey-finds-rising-misery-index-among-doctors/

4. Friedberg, M. et al., "Factors Affecting Physician Professional Satisfaction and Their Implications for Patient Care, Health Systems, and Health Policy," *Rand Corporation* 2013.

5. Ibid.

6. Jauhar, S., "Why Doctors Are Sick of Their Profession," *The Wall Street Journal*, August 29, 2014.

7. "Survey: Bureaucracy Crushing Texas Physicians," *Texas Medical Association*, December 4, 2014. http://www.texmed.org/Template.aspx?id=32469.

8. Babbott, S. et al., "Electronic Medical Records and Physician Stress in Primary Care: Results from the MEMO Study," *J Am Med Inform Assoc.*, 2014, 21: e100-e106. doi: 10.1136/amiajnl-2013-001875. Epub 2013 Sep 4.

9. Ibid.

10. Ibid.

Chapter 3:

1. Friedberg, M. et al., "Factors Affecting Physician Professional Satisfaction and Their Implications for Patient Care, Health Systems, and Health Policy," *Rand Corporation* 2013.

2. Drummond, D., *Stop Physician Burnout: What to Do When Working Harder Isn't Working* (Heritage Press Publications, LLC 2014).

3. Burch, N., "Four Stages for Learning Any New Skill," *Gordon Training International* 1970.

4. Jauhar, S., "Why Doctors Are Sick of Their Profession," *The Wall Street Journal*, August 29, 2014.

5. "You Can Afford Med School," *Association of American Medical Colleges*, May 2014.

6. Ibid.

7. Peckham, C., "Physician Burnout: It Just Keeps Getting Worse." *Medscape Physician Lifestyle Report* January 26, 2015.

8. Mayfield, T., "Photographer Captures Moment ER Doctor Steps Outside After Losing a 19-Year Old Patient," *Q13 Fox News*, March 19, 2015.

Chapter 4:

1. Rovner, J., "Medical Schools Reboot For 21st Century," *NPR*, April 9, 2015.

2. "Accelerating Change in Medical Education," *American Medical Association*, January 2013.

http://www.ama-assn.org/sub/accelerating-change/overview.shtml.

3. Beck, M., "Innovation is Sweeping Through U.S. Medical Schools," *The Wall Street Journal*, February 16, 2015.

4. Glicksman, E., "Wanting It All: A New Generation of Doctors Places Higher Value on Work-Life Balance," *Association of American Medical Colleges*, May 2013.

5. Ibid.

Chapter 5:

1. Shanafelt, TD. et al., "Impact of Organizational Leadership on Physician Burnout and Satisfaction," *Mayo Clinic Proceedings*, March 18, 2015.

2. Schoenbaum, S. et al., "Physicians' Views on Quality of Care: Findings From The Commonwealth Fund National Survey of Physicians and Quality of Care", *The Commonwealth Fund*, May 1, 2005.

3. Ibid.

4. Wilson Pecci, A., "Physician Burnout Heavily Influenced by Leadership Behaviors," *HealthLeaders Media*, April 28, 2015.

Chapter 6:

1. Shanafelt, TD. et al., "Burnout and Medical Errors Among American Surgeons," *Annals of Surgery*, 2010, 251 (6): 995-1000.

2. West, C. et al., "Association of Perceived Medical Errors With Resident Distress and Empathy," *JAMA*, 2006, 296 (9): 1071-1078.

3. Halbesleben, J. et al., "Linking Physician Burnout and Patient Outcomes: Exploring the Dyadic Relationship Between Physicians and Patients," *Health Care Management Review*, 2008, 33 (1): 29-39.

4. Doyle, C. et al., "A Systematic Review of Evidence on the Links Between Patient Experience and Clinical Safety and Effectiveness", *BMJ Open*, 2013; 3 e001570.

5. Curry, L., "What Distinguishes Top-Performing Hospitals in Acute Myocardial Infarction Mortality Rates," *Annals of Internal Medicine*, 2011, 154 (6): 384-390.

6. Haas, J. et al., "Is the Professional Satisfaction of General Internists Associated with Patient Satisfaction," *JGIM*, 2000, 15: 122-128.

7. DiMatteo, R. et al., "Physician's Characteristics Influence Patients' Adherence to Medical Treatment: Results From the Medical Outcomes Study," *Health Psychology*, 1993, 12 (2): 93-102.

8. Moyer. C., "Internist Attrition a Factor in Primary Care Physician Shortage," *American Medical News*, May 26, 2010.

9. Linzer, M., "Preventing Burnout in Academic Medicine," *Archives of Internal Medicine*, 2009, 169 (10): 927-928.

10. Walsh, K., "An Economic Argument for Investment in Physician Resilience", *Academic Medicine*, 2013, 88 (9): 1196.

11. Dewa, C. et al., "How does burnout affect physician productivity? A Systematic Literature Review," *BMC Health Services Research*, 2014, 14:325-34.

12. Rosin, T., "Bridging the Divide: How the Level of Physician Engagement Can Make or Break Your Hospital," *Becker's Hospital Review*, April 14, 2015.

13. Pearson, C. and Porath, C., *The Cost of Bad Behavior* (New York, Penguin Books, 2009).

14. Johnson, C., "Bad Blood: Doctor-Nurse Behavior Problems Impact Patient Care," *Physician Executive*, 32:696.

15. Jones, J. et al., "Stress and Medical Malpractice: Organizational Risk Assessment and Intervention," *Journal of Applied Psychology*, 1988, 73 (4):727-35.

16. Chen, Kuan-Yu et al., "Burnout, Job Satisfaction, and Medical Malpractice among Physicians," *International Journal of Medical Sciences*, 2013, 10 (11):1471-1478.

Chapter 7:

1. Wicks, R. J., *Overcoming Secondary Stress in Medical and Nursing Practice* (Oxford University Press, 2006) 18.

2. Mind Garden, http://www.mindgarden.com/117-maslach-burnout-inventory.

3. Shelton, A., *Transforming Burnout: A Simple Guide to Self-Renewal* (Vibrant Press, 2007) p. 9.

4. Wallace, J. et al., "Physician Wellness: A Missing Quality Indicator," *The Lancet*, November 2009, vol. 374 (9702):1714-21.

5. Lindeman, S. et al., "A systematic review on gender-specific suicide mortality in medical doctors," *Br J Psychiatry*, March 1996, 168 (3):274-9.

6. American Foundation for Suicide Prevention, https://www.afsp.org/preventing-suicide/suicide-warning-signs

Chapter 10:

1. Nelson, B., "The Ten Ironies of Motivation," *Workforce*, February 1, 1999.

Chapter 11:

1. Rosenstein, A., "Physician Stress and Burnout: What Can We Do," *Physician Executive Journal*, 2012, Nov-Dec: 22-30.

2. Institute of Medicine, Education, and Spirituality, http://www.ochsner.org/imeso

Chapter 12:

1. Howlett M. et al., "Burnout in Emergency Department Healthcare Professionals is Associated with Coping Style: A Cross-Sectional Survey," *Emergency Medicine Journal*, 2015, 0:1-6.

2. Sinha, P., "Why Do Doctors Commit Suicide," *The New York Times*, September 4, 2014.

3. Peckham, C., "Medscape Physician Lifestyle Report 2015: Physician Burnout and Vacation Time," *Medscape*, January 26, 2015.

4. Jensen, P. et al., "Building Physician Resilience," *Can Fam Physician*, May 2008, 54(5):722-29.

5. Fitch, S., "5 Ways to Use Creativity to Combat Physician Burnout," *Love Medicine Again*, April 14, 2015.

6. Leebov, W., *Essentials for Great Patient Experiences* (American Hospital Association, April 2008).

7. Peckham, C., "Medscape Physician Lifestyle Report 2015: Physician Burnout and Volunteer Time," *Medscape*, January 26, 2015.

8. Horoszowski, M., "5 Surprising Benefits of Volunteering," *Forbes*, March 19, 2015.

9. Peckham, C., "Medscape Physician Lifestyle Report 2015: Do Burned-Out Physicians Have Less in Savings," *Medscape*, January 26, 2015.

10. Kabat-Zinn, J., *Wherever You Go There You Are* (New York, Hyperion, 2005).

ADDITIONAL RESOURCES

ABOUT STUDER GROUP®, A HURON HEALTHCARE SOLUTION:

Learn more about Studer Group® by scanning the QR code with your mobile device or by visiting www. studergroup.com/who-we-are/about-studer-group.

Studer Group works with healthcare organizations in the United States, Canada, Australia, and beyond to help them achieve and sustain exceptional improvement in clinical outcomes and financial results. A Huron Healthcare solution, Studer Group partners with organizations to build a sustainable culture that promotes accountability, fosters innovation, and consistently delivers a great patient experience and the best quality outcomes over time. By installing an execution framework called Evidence-Based Leadership^{SM} (EBL), organizations are able to align goals, actions, and processes and execute quickly. This framework creates the foundation that enables transformation in this era of continuous change.

To learn more about partnering with Studer Group on your journey to improvement, visit www.studergroup.com or call 850-439-5839.

STUDER GROUP COACHING:

Learn more about Studer Group coaching by scanning the QR code with your mobile device or by visiting www.studergroup.com/coaching.

Studer Group coaches partner with healthcare organizations to create an aligned culture accountable to achieving outcomes together. Working side-by-side, we help to establish, accelerate, and hardwire the necessary changes to create a culture of excellence. This leads to better transparency, higher accountability, and the ability to target and execute specific, objective results that organizations want to achieve.

System Coaching Partnership

As systems today are looking to meet the challenges of the external environment and mergers and acquisitions are more and more common, it's critical to align operations to create a feeling of cultural integration and standardize this approach. We do this by coaching leaders and their teams on how to hardwire evidence-based tools and processes that have been proven to accelerate and sustain performance improvement across the board, especially operational, clinical, and service excellence. We work to align organization leaders from the top down, to focus on the outcomes that really matter to long-term success. Creating consistency across the organization and putting in place systems of accountability are crucial to executing operational and strategic plans.

Evidence-Based Leadership^{SM} (EBL) Coaching

There are plenty of tools and tactics proven to improve clinical quality, patient perception of care, and, yes, profitability. Yet no matter how many an organization implements, without the right foundation in place, any bursts of improvement will be sporadic and short-lived.

That's why Studer Group helps partner organizations install a framework called Evidence-Based Leadership (EBL). This framework aligns organizational goals, behaviors, and processes in a way that moves and sustains results. Combined with a set of proven tactics and best practices refined in our National Learning Lab consisting of hundreds of hospitals, EBL empowers our partners to hardwire profitability into every corner of their organization—and, ultimately, to succeed in the pay-for-performance era.

Specialized Emergency Department Coaching Partnership

With public reporting of data coming in the future, healthcare organizations can no longer accept crowded Emergency Departments and long patient wait times. Studer Group's Emergency Department coaching division provides evidence-based best practices and tools that help EDs execute results. Through research-supported tools and tactics and executive leadership coaching, Studer Group ED experts work to create alignment from the executive team to the frontline leaders. We are able to diagnose areas of opportunity from the start, such as flow and throughput issues, that not only benefit the ED but positively affect the results of the entire organization.

Physician Coaching Partnership

Studer Group's physician coaching helps organizations integrate and partner with their physicians. From an initial survey and needs assessment, a comprehensive physician coaching plan and strategy is developed. With the support of their coaching team, physician leaders implement Studer Group's proven tools and tactics to improve physician alignment and engagement, which leads to improved quality, safety, and patient perception of care. Physician coaching supports organizational priorities while ensuring that physician engagement and culture thrive. It also provides development to close metric gaps and further develop physician skills to improve outcomes for patients.

Medical Practice Coaching Partnership

Medical practice coaching provides evidence-based tools and tactics that help those in an ambulatory setting achieve and sustain results. Our medical practice experts provide the structure and framework that allows practices to adapt to change quickly. Studer Group's Evidence-Based Leadership framework, paired with onsite coaching and resources specially designed and tested in the outpatient setting, allows practices to truly transform. We are able to tailor our approach and drive results across all pillars to positively impact the pillars and hardwire profitability.

Rural Healthcare Coaching Partnership

The changes in healthcare demand constant, unrelenting improvement and the ability to do more with less. That's true whether you're a 1,000-bed system or a 50-bed community hospital. However, if you're the latter, your less is considerably less than their less. You need to create a culture of high performance that aligns your entire organization and allows you to achieve and sustain high-level quality outcomes—and you need to do it in a way that your resources will allow.

Studer Group's Rural Partnership focuses our intellectual resources and Evidence-Based Leadership framework to meet your particular set of needs. In addition to other benefits, rural partners gain access to our performance expert coaches and the proven tools and best practices from our National Learning Lab consisting of hundreds of hospitals.

BOOKS: CATEGORIZED BY AUDIENCE

Explore the Fire Starter Publishing website by scanning the QR code with your mobile device or by visiting www.firestarterpublishing.com.

Senior Leaders & Physicians

A Culture of High Performance: Achieving Higher Quality at a Lower Cost—A must-have book for any leader struggling to shore up margins while sustaining an organization that is a great place for employees to work, physicians to practice medicine, and patients to receive care. From best-selling author Quint Studer to help you build a culture that will thrive during change.

Straight A Leadership: Alignment, Action, Accountability—A guide that will help you identify gaps in alignment, action, and accountability; create a plan to fill them; and become a more resourceful, agile, high-performing organization, written by Quint Studer.

Engaging Physicians: A Manual to Physician Partnership—A tactical and passionate road map for physician collaboration to generate organizational high performance, written by Stephen C. Beeson, MD.

Excellence with an Edge: Practicing Medicine in a Competitive Environment—An insightful book that provides practical tools and techniques you need to know to have a solid grasp of the business side of making a living in healthcare, written by Michael T. Harris, MD.

Physicians

The CG CAHPS Handbook: A Guide to Improve Patient Experience and Clinical Outcomes—Written by Jeff Morris, MD, MBA, FACS; Barbara Hotko, RN, MPA; and Matthew Bates, MPH. *The CG CAHPS Handbook* is your guide for consistently delivering on what matters most to patients and their families and for providing exceptional care and improved clinical outcomes.

Practicing Excellence: A Physician's Manual to Exceptional Health Care—This book, written by Stephen C. Beeson, MD, is a brilliant guide to implementing physician leadership and behaviors that will create a high-performance workplace.

All Leaders

101 Answers to Questions Leaders Ask—By Quint Studer and Studer Group coaches, offers practical, prescriptive solutions from healthcare leaders around the country.

Eat That Cookie!: Make Workplace Positivity Pay Off...For Individuals, Teams, and Organizations—Written by Liz Jazwiec, RN, this book is funny, inspiring, relatable, and is packed with realistic, down-to-earth tactics to infuse positivity into your culture.

Hardwiring Excellence—A *BusinessWeek* bestseller, this book is a road map to creating and sustaining a "Culture of Service and Operational Excellence" that drives bottom-line results. Written by Quint Studer.

Hey Cupcake! We Are ALL Leaders—Author Liz Jazwiec explains that we'll all eventually be called on to lead someone, whether it's a department, a shift, a project team, or a new employee. In her trademark slightly sarcastic (and hilarious) voice, she provides learned-the-hard-way insights that will benefit leaders in every industry and at every level.

"I'm Sorry to Hear That..." Real-Life Responses to Patients' 101 Most Common Complaints About Health Care—When you respond to a patient's complaint, you are responding to the patient's sense of helplessness and anxiety. The service recovery scripts offered in this book can help you recover a patient's confidence in you and your organization. Authored by Susan Keane Baker and Leslie Bank.

Oh No...Not More of That Fluffy Stuff! The Power of Engagement—Written by Rich Bluni, RN, this funny, heartfelt book explores what it takes to overcome obstacles and tap into the passion that fuels our best work. Its practical exercises help employees at all levels get happier, more excited, and more connected to the meaning in our daily lives.

Over Our Heads: An Analogy on Healthcare, Good Intentions, and Unforeseen Consequences—This book, written by Rulon F. Stacey, PhD, FACHE, uses a grocery store analogy to illustrate how government intervention leads to economic crisis and, eventually, collapse.

Results That Last: Hardwiring Behaviors That Will Take Your Company to the Top—A *Wall Street Journal* bestseller by Quint Studer that teaches leaders in every industry how to apply his tactics and strategies to their own organizations to build a corporate culture that consistently reaches and exceeds its goals.

Service Excellence Is As Easy As PIE (Perception Is Everything)—Realistic, down to earth, and wickedly witty, *PIE* is perfect for everyone in healthcare or any other service industry. It's filled with ideas for creating exceptional customer experiences—ideas that are surprising, simple, and yes, easy as you-know-what. Written by Liz Jazwiec.

The Great Employee Handbook: Making Work and Life Better—This book is a valuable resource for employees at all levels who want to learn how to handle tough workplace situations—skills that normally come only from a lifetime of experience. *Wall Street Journal* best-selling author Quint Studer has pulled together the best insights gained from working with thousands of employees during his career.

Nurse Leaders and Nurses

Inspired Nurse and *Inspired Journal*—By Rich Bluni, RN, help maintain and recapture the inspiration nurses felt at the start of their journey with action-oriented "spiritual stretches" and stories that illuminate those sacred moments we all experience.

The HCAHPS Handbook, 2nd Edition: Tactics to Improve Quality and the Patient Experience—Revised and released in 2015, this book is a valuable resource for organizations seeking to provide the exceptional quality of care their patients expect and deserve. Coauthored by Lyn Ketelsen, RN, MBA; Karen Cook, RN; and Bekki Kennedy.

The Nurse Leader Handbook: The Art and Science of Nurse Leadership—By Studer Group senior nursing and physician leaders from across the country, is filled with knowledge that provides nurse leaders with a solid foundation for success. It also serves as a reference they can revisit again and again when they have questions or need a quick refresher course in a particular area of the job.

Emergency Department Team

Advance Your Emergency Department: Leading in a New Era—As this critical book asserts, world-class Emergency Departments don't follow. They lead. Stephanie J. Baker, RN, CEN, MBA; Regina Shupe, RN, MSN, CEN; and Dan Smith, MD, FACEP, share high-impact strategies and tactics to help your ED get results more efficiently, effectively, and collaboratively. Master them and you'll improve quality, exceed patient expectations, and ultimately help the entire organization maintain and grow its profit margin.

Excellence in the Emergency Department: How to Get Results—A book by Stephanie Baker, RN, CEN, MBA, is filled with proven, easy-to-implement, step-by-step instructions that will help you move your Emergency Department forward.

Hardwiring Flow: Systems and Processes for Seamless Patient Care—Drs. Thom Mayer and Kirk Jensen delve into one of the most critical issues facing healthcare leaders: patient flow.

The Patient Flow Advantage: How Hardwiring Hospital-Wide Flow Drives Competitive Performance—Build effectiveness, efficiency, and a patient-centric focus into the heart of every process that serves the patient. Efficient patient flow has never been more critical to ensure patient safety, satisfaction, and optimal reimbursement. Authored by Drs. Kirk Jensen and Thom Mayer.

STUDER CONFERENCES:

Learn more about Studer Group conferences by scanning the QR code with your mobile device or by visiting www.studergroup.com/conferences.

Studer Conferences are three-day interactive learning events designed to provide healthcare leaders with an authentic, practical learning experience.

Each Studer Conference includes internationally renowned keynote speakers and tracks concentrated on key areas of the healthcare organization. Every track includes breakout sessions and "how-to" workshops that provide you with direct access to experts and conference faculty. The faculty at Studer Conferences go beyond PowerPoint slides and lectures to show you "what right looks like."

Leaders will leave with new tools and skills that get results. Find out more about upcoming Studer Conferences and register at www.studergroup.com/conferences.

All Studer Group Conferences offer Continuing Education Credits. For more information on CMEs, visit www.studergroup.com/cmecredits.

About the Author

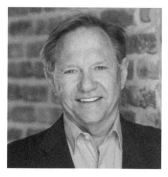

Quint Studer is the founder of Studer Group®, a Huron Healthcare solution. A recipient of the 2010 Malcolm Baldrige National Quality Award, Studer Group is an outcomes firm that implements Evidence-Based Leadership℠ systems and practices to help organizations achieve, sustain, and accelerate performance in service, quality, finance, people, and growth.

Studer has been in the healthcare field for over 31 years and spends much of his time creating and sharing best practices with hundreds of healthcare professionals each month. A frequent keynoter at national and organization events, he regularly meets with healthcare leaders around the country at client engagements and Studer Group-sponsored institutes. He is also a frequently interviewed healthcare leader in the national media.

Inc. magazine named Studer its Master of Business, making him the only healthcare leader to have ever won this award. Twice, *Modern Healthcare* has chosen him as one of the 100 Most Powerful People in Healthcare. In March 2014, he was also named one of the 40 Smartest People in Healthcare Today by *Becker's Hospital Review*. In September of 2014, he was the first ever recipient of *Modern Healthcare's* Healthcare Marketing Visionary IMPACT Award. Studer is currently part of the 21st Healthcare Leadership Curriculum Task Force at Harvard Business School. He has served as a board member at the Association of University Programs in Health Administration (AUPHA) and the Healthcare Financial Management Association (HFMA). He has also served as a think tank panelist in Washington, D.C., and is faculty in residence at George Washington University and a guest professor at Cornell University. He currently serves on the board of a major healthcare system. In addition, he serves as an entrepreneur in residence at the Center for Entrepreneurship at the University of West Florida, College of Business.

Besides *Healing Physician Burnout*, Studer has written and contributed to a number of books. *Maximize Performance* was written for education and was just released in January 2015. *A Culture of High Performance*, released in 2013, helps organizations achieve higher quality at a lower cost. His first book, *Hardwiring Excellence*, a *BusinessWeek* bestseller, is one of the most-read leadership books ever written for healthcare. More than 700,000 copies are in circulation. His book *Results That Last* hit the *Wall Street Journal's* bestseller list of business books.

Straight A Leadership provides a methodology for organizations to assess their alignment, action, and accountability. One of his most popular books, *The Great Employee Handbook*, provides actions employees can take to better not only their work, but their lives as well.

In his latest book, *Healing Physician Burnout*, Studer offers tactics organizations can use to help create a better work environment for physicians as they deal with major industry changes. He also identifies signs and symptoms of burnout so that leaders can recognize it in physicians—and physicians can recognize it in themselves—in order to seek help and healing early on.

How to Order Additional Copies of

Healing Physician Burnout: Diagnosing, Preventing, and Treating

Orders may be placed:

Online at:
www.firestarterpublishing.com/healingphysicianburnout

Scan the QR code with your mobile device to order through
the Fire Starter Publishing website.

By phone at: 866-354-3473

By mail at: Fire Starter Publishing
913 Gulf Breeze Parkway, Suite 6
Gulf Breeze, FL 32561

Share this book with your team—and save!
Healing Physician Burnout: Diagnosing, Preventing, and Treating
is filled with valuable information. That's why we're of-
fering bulk discounts when you order multiple copies.
(The more you order, the more you save!)
For details, see www.firestarterpublishing.com.